LOW-CARB VEGETARIAN DIET COOKBOOK
FOR BEGINNERS

The Beginner-Friendly Guide with 50 Nutritious, Quick & Easy Low-Sugar, Plant-Based Recipes for Sustaining Vitality and Wellbeing

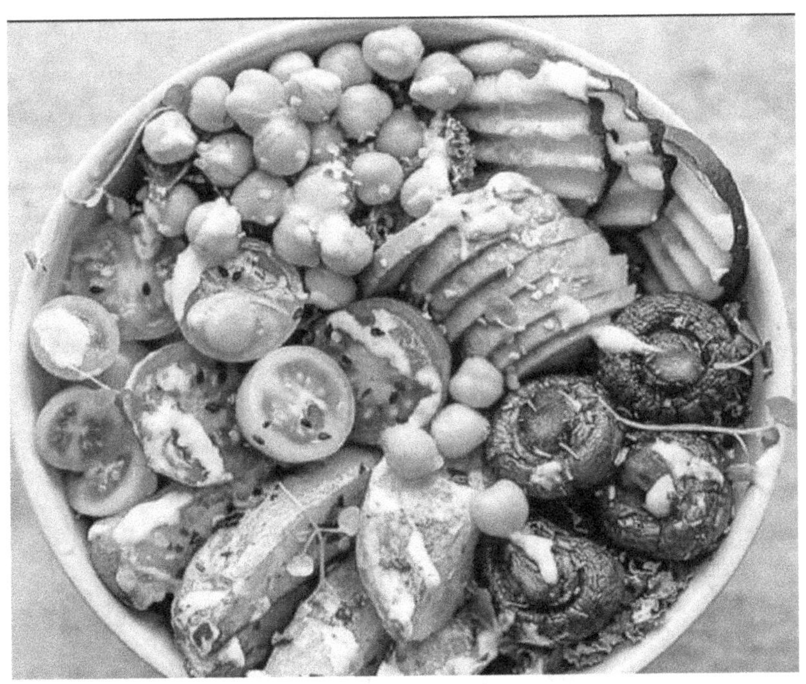

DR. COLE HULL

COPYRIGHT

All rights reserved. No part of this publication may be reproduced, stored in a retrieval system, or transmitted in any form or by any means, electronic, mechanical, photocopying, recording, or otherwise, without the prior written permission of the author, except for brief quotations in critical reviews or articles.

COPYRIGHT © 2024 BY DR. COLE HULL

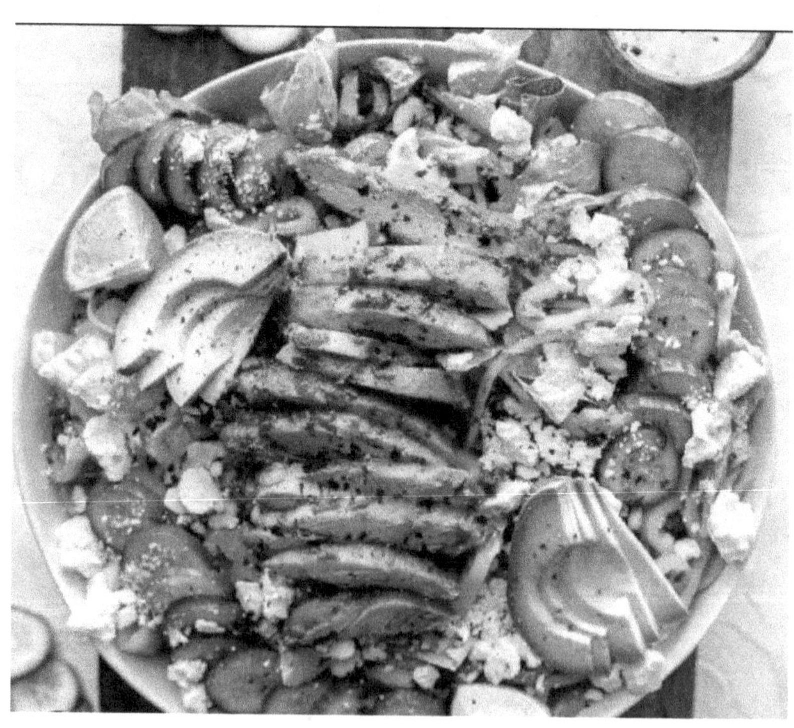

TABLE OF CONTENT

INTRODUCTION 7

Understanding Low-Carb Vegetarian Basics........................ 8

Shopping List for a Low-Carb Vegetarian Pantry 11

CHAPTER 1: BREAKFASTS... 15

1. Chia and Almond Milk Porridge................................. 15

2. Spinach and Mushroom Omelet Cups 17

3. Keto Avocado Smoothie with Coconut Milk.................. 19

4. Low-Carb Blueberry Muffins (Almond Flour)................ 20

5. Shakshuka with Feta (No Bread) 23

6. Cauliflower and Cheese Breakfast Muffins 25

7. Almond and Flaxseed Pancakes................................. 27

8. Coconut Yogurt with Nuts and Seeds 30

9. Bell Pepper and Kale Frittata.................................... 32

10. Pumpkin Spice Chia Pudding 34

CHAPTER 2: LUNCHES.. 37

11. Zucchini Noodles with Avocado Pesto...................... 37

12. Cauliflower Tabouleh 39

13. Creamy Spinach Soup (Dairy-Free)......................... 41

14. Greek Salad with Tofu Feta 43

15. Caprese Stuffed Avocado 45

16. Broccoli and Almond Salad 47

17. Keto Eggplant Pizza Rounds 49

18. Cucumber Boat with Spicy Tofu Salad 51

19. Asparagus and Artichoke Heart Salad 53

20. Roasted Red Pepper and Goat Cheese Zucchini Rolls ... 55

CHAPTER 3: DINNERS 59

21. Mushroom Stroganoff (Zucchini Noodles)..................... 59

22. Cauliflower Steak with Chimichurri Sauce 61

23. Spaghetti Squash with Creamy Mushroom Sauce 64

24. Baked Tofu with Peanut Sauce and Stir-Fry Veggies 66

25. Grilled Halloumi with Mediterranean Vegetables.......... 69

26. Vegan Alfredo with Shirataki Noodles.......................... 71

27. Vegetable Korma (Cauliflower Rice) 73

28. Stuffed Bell Peppers (Quinoa and Vegetables) 76

29. Paneer Tikka Skewers.. 78

30. Moroccan Tagine with Turnip and Zucchini 81

CHAPTER 4: SNACKS AND SIDES 85

31. Avocado and Walnut Salad.................................... 85

32. Keto Garlic Bread Sticks (Cauliflower Base)............... 87

33. Marinated Artichoke Hearts.................................... 89

34. Roasted Brussels Sprouts with Pecans........................ 91

35. Eggplant Dip (Baba Ganoush) 93

36. Vegan Cheese (Nut-Based)..................................... 95

37. Spicy Pumpkin Seeds.. 97

38. Zucchini Chips 99

39. Olive and Tomato Tapenade................................... 101

40. Creamy Cucumber Salad with Dill 102

CHAPTER 5: DESSERTS AND DRINKS 105

41. Blackberry and Mint Infused Water 105

42. Coconut and Raspberry Keto Fat............................. 106

43. Almond Butter and Chocolate Fudge 108

44. Lemon Cheesecake Mousse (Sugar-Free) 110

45. Strawberries Dipped in Vegan Dark Chocolate............... 112

46. Matcha Chia Seed Pudding................................... 114

47. Pumpkin Pie Smoothie (Dairy-Free) 116

48. Keto Avocado Popsicles 118

49. Cinnamon and Pecan Porridge (Flaxseed Meal)............... 120

50. Ginger and Lemon Hot Tea (Sweetened with Stevia) .. 122

CHAPTER 6: 14-DAY LOW-CARB VEGETARIAN MEAL PLAN 125

CONCLUSION 131

Tips for Long-Term Success on a Low-Carb Vegetarian Diet 131

How to Adapt and Personalize Recipes for Your Needs 132

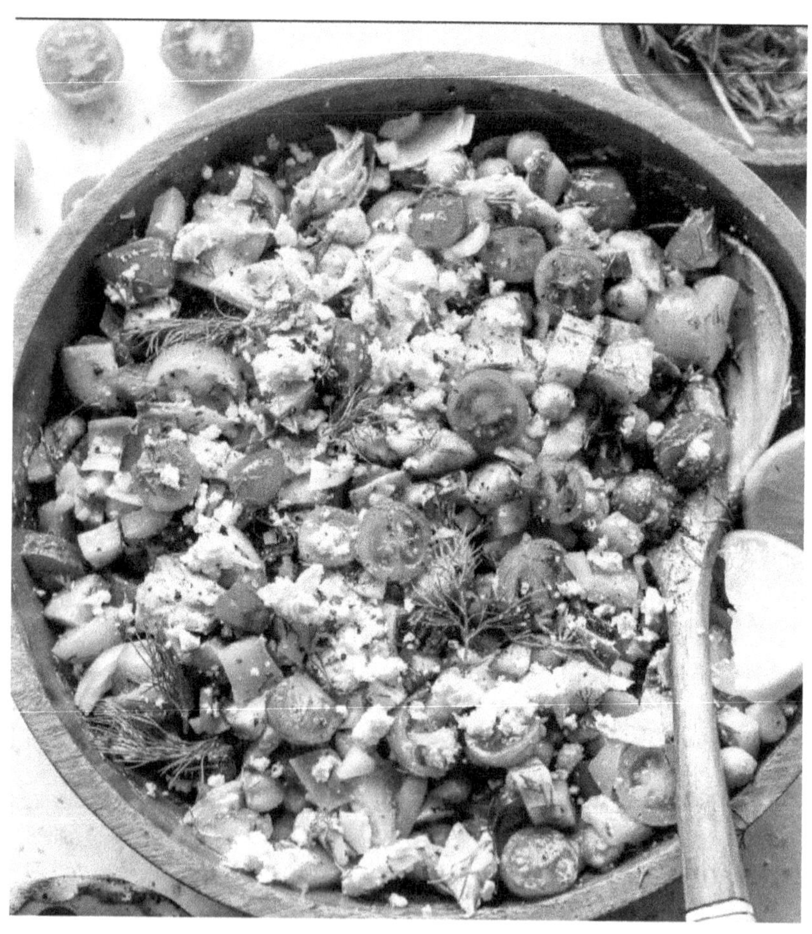

INTRODUCTION

Embarking on a journey into low-carb vegetarian eating is a transformative step towards embracing a healthier lifestyle that benefits both mind and body. This dietary approach combines the principles of reducing carbohydrate intake with a vegetarian lifestyle, focusing on whole foods to nourish your body while minimizing processed foods and sugars. This way of eating not only supports weight management but also enhances overall well-being, offering a sustainable path to long-term health.

Adopting a low-carb vegetarian diet doesn't mean sacrificing flavor or variety. Instead, it opens up a world of culinary creativity, encouraging the exploration of diverse vegetables, healthy fats, and plant-based proteins. This diet emphasizes nutrient-dense foods that are naturally low in carbs, such as leafy greens, nuts, seeds, and certain dairy products, allowing you to enjoy satisfying meals that align with your health goals.

As you begin this journey, remember that the transition to a low-carb vegetarian lifestyle is a personal experience, unique to each individual's tastes, preferences, and nutritional needs. This book is designed to guide you through the basics, offering delicious, easy-to-prepare recipes that make it simple to stick to your low-carb vegetarian goals. Whether you're a seasoned vegetarian looking to reduce carb intake or you're new to this way of eating, our goal is to provide you with the knowledge, inspiration, and tools needed to succeed.

Welcome to a world of vibrant flavors, fresh ingredients, and healthful eating. Let's embark on this delicious journey together.

Understanding Low-Carb Vegetarian Basics

Transitioning to a low-carb vegetarian diet involves more than just reducing your intake of carbohydrates; it's about making informed choices to ensure your meals are nutritious, satisfying, and aligned with vegetarian principles. At its core, a low-carb vegetarian diet aims to limit high-carb foods like sugars, grains, and starchy vegetables, focusing instead on protein sources, non-starchy vegetables, and healthy fats.

Key Components of a Low-Carb Vegetarian Diet:

- **Proteins:** Protein is crucial for building and repairing tissues, among other vital functions. In a low-carb vegetarian diet, protein sources include dairy products (for lacto-vegetarians), eggs (for ovo-vegetarians), and a variety of plant-based proteins such as tofu, tempeh, seitan, legumes, and nuts. These foods provide essential amino acids, the building blocks of protein, which are necessary for health.

- **Fats:** Healthy fats are a cornerstone of the low-carb vegetarian diet, providing energy, supporting cell function, and helping with the absorption of vitamins. Sources of healthy fats include avocados, olive oil, coconut oil, nuts, seeds, and full-fat dairy products. These fats can help you feel full and satisfied while ensuring your diet is flavorful and diverse.

- **Carbohydrates:** While following a low-carb diet, it's important to choose your carbs wisely. Focus on fiber-rich, nutrient-dense vegetables such as leafy greens (spinach, kale, and arugula), cruciferous vegetables (broccoli, cauliflower, and Brussels sprouts), and other non-starchy vegetables. These foods provide essential vitamins, minerals, and fiber, which can help maintain digestive health and stabilize blood sugar levels.

- **Vitamins and Minerals:** A well-planned low-carb vegetarian diet should also include foods rich in vitamins and minerals to ensure nutritional adequacy. This includes a variety of vegetables, nuts, seeds, and fortified foods to cover nutrients that may be more challenging to obtain, such as Vitamin B12, Iron, Calcium, and Omega-3 fatty acids.

Balancing Your Meals:

Creating balanced meals on a low-carb vegetarian diet involves combining protein, fats, and low-carb vegetables to ensure you're getting a wide range of nutrients while staying within your carb limit. It's also important to listen to your body and adjust your food choices based on your energy needs, health goals, and how you feel.

Understanding these basics sets the foundation for a successful low-carb vegetarian lifestyle. With this knowledge, you can confidently navigate your dietary choices, ensuring they are both enjoyable and in line with your health objectives.

Shopping List for a Low-Carb Vegetarian Pantry

Equipping your pantry and refrigerator with the right ingredients is the first step to successfully adopting a low-carb vegetarian lifestyle. Having a variety of essential items on hand makes meal preparation easier, ensures your meals are nutritious and helps you stay on track with your dietary goals. Below is a comprehensive shopping list designed to cover the basics of low-carb vegetarian eating, making it simple to create delicious, healthful meals at home.

Vegetables:

- Leafy greens (spinach, kale, lettuce)
- Cruciferous vegetables (broccoli, cauliflower, Brussels sprouts)
- Zucchini
- Bell peppers
- Mushrooms
- Avocados
- Asparagus
- Eggplant
- Cucumbers
- Tomatoes (moderately, due to higher carb content)

Fruits (Low-Carb Options):

- Berries (strawberries, raspberries, blackberries, in moderation)
- Lemons and limes

Proteins:

- Eggs
- Dairy (cheese, Greek yogurt, butter, heavy cream for those who include dairy)
- Tofu
- Tempeh
- Seitan (note: check carb content, as it can vary)
- Plant-based protein powders (pea, hemp, or rice protein)

Healthy Fats:

- Nuts (almonds, walnuts, pecans, macadamia nuts)
- Seeds (chia, flaxseed, pumpkin seeds, sunflower seeds)
- Olive oil
- Coconut oil
- Avocado oil
- Full-fat coconut milk

Pantry Staples:

- Almond flour
- Coconut flour
- Flax meal
- Unsweetened cocoa powder
- Low-carb sweeteners (stevia, erythritol, monk fruit sweetener)
- Soy sauce or tamari (gluten-free)
- Nutritional yeast
- Vegetable broth (low sodium)
- Canned tomatoes (no added sugar)
- Olives
- Pickles (no added sugar)

Herbs and Spices:

- Fresh herbs (cilantro, parsley, basil)
- Dried spices (turmeric, cumin, paprika, chili powder)
- Salt and pepper
- Garlic
- Ginger

Condiments:

- Mustard

- Vinegar (apple cider, balsamic, red wine)

- Hot sauce

- Salsa (check for added sugars)

This list is a starting point, meant to be adapted based on personal preferences, nutritional needs, and specific dietary restrictions. By stocking your kitchen with these ingredients, you'll be well-prepared to explore the variety of flavors and textures that low-carb vegetarian cooking has to offer. Remember, the key to a successful and satisfying diet is variety, so don't hesitate to try new foods and experiment with different recipes.

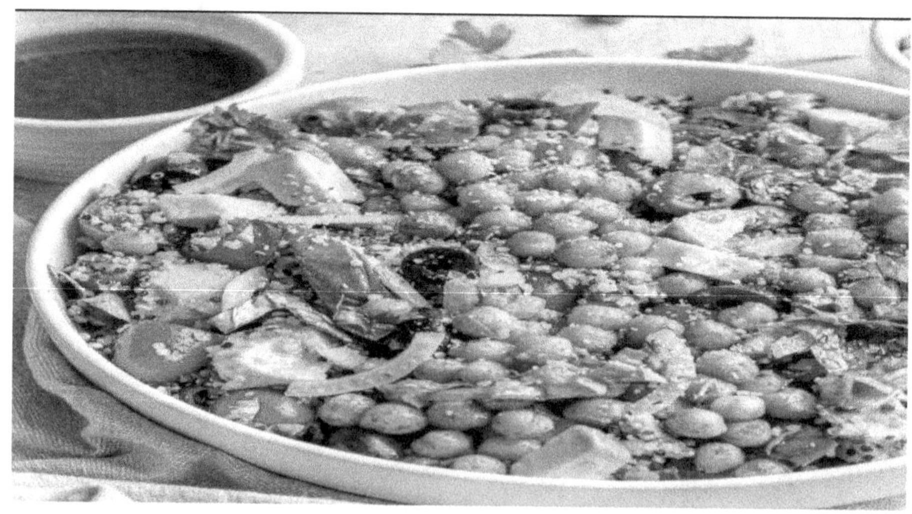

1. Chia and Almond Milk Porridge

Prep time: 5 minutes

Cook time: 0 minutes (requires overnight refrigeration)

Serving size: 2 servings

Ingredients:

- 1/4 cup chia seeds

- 1 cup unsweetened almond milk

- 1/2 teaspoon vanilla extract

- 1 tablespoon sugar-free maple syrup or sweetener of choice

- 1/4 teaspoon cinnamon

- Optional toppings: sliced almonds, berries, and a dollop of almond butter

Nutritional facts (per serving, without toppings):

- Calories: 150

- Carbohydrates: 12g

- Fiber: 9g

- Protein: 5g

- Fat: 9g

Preparation directions:

1. In a bowl, mix chia seeds, almond milk, vanilla extract, sweetener, and cinnamon.
2. Stir the mixture thoroughly to ensure the chia seeds are well dispersed and starting to gel.
3. Cover the bowl and refrigerate overnight, or at least for 6 hours.
4. Before serving, stir the porridge well. If it's too thick, add a bit more almond milk to reach your desired consistency.
5. Serve with optional toppings like sliced almonds, berries, or almond butter for added flavor and nutrients.

Health benefit:

This Chia and Almond Milk Porridge is a fantastic low-carb, high-fiber breakfast option for vegetarians. The chia seeds are an excellent source of omega-3 fatty acids, antioxidants, and minerals such as calcium and magnesium, supporting heart health and bone strength. The high fiber content aids in digestion and helps maintain stable blood sugar levels, making it an ideal start to the day for energy and satiety.

2. Spinach and Mushroom Omelet Cups

Prep time: 10 minutes

Cook time: 20 minutes

Serving size: 6 omelet cups

Ingredients:

- 6 large eggs

- 1/2 cup chopped fresh spinach

- 1/2 cup diced mushrooms

- 1/4 cup diced onions

- 1/4 cup shredded cheese (cheddar or mozzarella)

- Salt and pepper to taste

- 1 tablespoon olive oil

Nutritional facts (per omelet cup):

- Calories: 110 kcal

- Carbohydrates: 2g

- Fiber: 0.5g

- Protein: 7g

- Fat: 8g

Preparation directions:

1. Preheat the oven to 350°F (175°C). Grease a muffin tin with olive oil.
2. Heat a skillet over medium heat. Add olive oil, onions, mushrooms, and spinach. Sauté until the vegetables are soft, about 5 minutes.
3. In a large bowl, whisk the eggs. Stir in the cooked vegetables and shredded cheese. Season with salt and pepper.
4. Divide the mixture evenly among the muffin tin cups.
5. Bake in the preheated oven for 20 minutes, or until the eggs are set.
6. Allow to cool for a few minutes before removing from the muffin tin.

Health benefit:

Spinach and Mushroom Omelet Cups offer a protein-rich, nutrient-dense start to the day. Eggs provide a high-quality protein source, essential for muscle repair and growth, while spinach contributes iron and vitamins A and C, crucial for energy production and immune support. Mushrooms add a boost of antioxidants and B vitamins, supporting brain health and energy metabolism. This combination makes for a balanced, healthful breakfast option for vegetarians.

3. Keto Avocado Smoothie with Coconut Milk

Prep time: 5 minutes

Serving size: 1 serving

Ingredients:

- 1/2 ripe avocado

- 1 cup unsweetened coconut milk

- 1/4 teaspoon vanilla extract

- Sweetener to taste (e.g., stevia or erythritol)

- Ice cubes (optional)

Nutritional facts (per serving):

- Calories: 300 kcal

- Carbohydrates: 8g

- Fiber: 5g

- Protein: 3g

- Fat: 29g

Preparation directions:

1. Scoop the avocado flesh into a blender.

2. Add the coconut milk, vanilla extract, sweetener, and ice cubes if using.

3. Blend on high until smooth and creamy.

4. Taste and adjust sweetness if necessary.

5. Serve immediately for the best flavor and texture.

Health benefit:

The Keto Avocado Smoothie with Coconut Milk is an excellent low-carb breakfast choice, providing healthy fats from both avocado and coconut milk. Avocados are rich in monounsaturated fats, which are beneficial for heart health and skin health. Coconut milk contributes to healthy fat intake, helping to increase satiety and provide energy. This smoothie is also hydrating and contains essential vitamins and minerals, supporting overall health and well-being for vegetarians.

4. Low-Carb Blueberry Muffins (Almond Flour)

Prep time: 10 minutes

Cook time: 25 minutes

Serving size: 12 muffins

Ingredients:

- 2 cups almond flour

- 1/2 cup erythritol (or another low-carb sweetener)

- 1 teaspoon baking powder

- 1/4 teaspoon salt

- 3 large eggs

- 1/3 cup unsweetened almond milk

- 1/4 cup melted coconut oil

- 1 teaspoon vanilla extract

- 1/2 cup fresh or frozen blueberries

Nutritional facts (per muffin):

- Calories: 160 kcal

- Carbohydrates: 6g

- Fiber: 3g

- Protein: 5g

- Fat: 14g

Preparation directions:

1. Preheat your oven to 350°F (175°C) and line a muffin tin with paper liners or grease with coconut oil.

2. In a large bowl, mix together the almond flour, erythritol, baking powder, and salt.

3. In another bowl, whisk together the eggs, almond milk, melted coconut oil, and vanilla extract.

4. Combine the wet and dry ingredients until just mixed. Gently fold in the blueberries.

5. Divide the batter evenly among the muffin cups, filling each about 3/4 full.

6. Bake for 25 minutes, or until the tops are golden and a toothpick inserted into the center comes out clean.

7. Let the muffins cool in the pan for 5 minutes before transferring them to a wire rack to cool completely.

Health benefit:

Low-Carb Blueberry Muffins made with almond flour are an excellent breakfast option for vegetarians looking to maintain a low-carb diet. Almond flour provides a gluten-free alternative to traditional flour, rich in protein, fiber, and healthy fats, especially vitamin E, an antioxidant that supports skin health. Blueberries add a burst of flavor and antioxidants, such as vitamin C and K, fiber, and phytonutrients, supporting heart health and providing anti-inflammatory benefits.

5. Shakshuka with Feta (No Bread)

Prep time: 10 minutes

Cook time: 20 minutes

Serving size: 4 servings

Ingredients:

- 1 tablespoon olive oil

- 1/2 cup diced onions

- 1 bell pepper, diced

- 2 cloves garlic, minced

- 1 teaspoon paprika

- 1/2 teaspoon cumin

- 1/4 teaspoon chili powder (optional)

- 1 can (14 oz) diced tomatoes, no sugar added

- Salt and pepper to taste

- 4 large eggs

- 1/2 cup crumbled feta cheese

- Fresh cilantro or parsley for garnish

Nutritional facts (per serving):

- Calories: 180 kcal

- Carbohydrates: 9g

- Fiber: 2g

- Protein: 10g

- Fat: 12g

Preparation directions:

1. Heat olive oil in a large skillet over medium heat. Add onions and bell pepper, cooking until softened, about 5 minutes.

2. Add garlic, paprika, cumin, and chili powder, cooking for another minute until fragrant.

3. Pour in the diced tomatoes (with juices), season with salt and pepper, and simmer for 10 minutes until the sauce thickens slightly.

4. Make four wells in the sauce with a spoon. Crack an egg into each well.

5. Cover the skillet and cook until the eggs are just set, about 7-10 minutes.

6. Sprinkle crumbled feta cheese over the top and garnish with fresh cilantro or parsley.

7. Serve hot, directly from the skillet.

Health benefit:

Shakshuka with Feta is a flavorful and nutritious low-carb breakfast option, providing a good balance of proteins, healthy fats, and vitamins. Eggs are a complete protein source, containing all nine essential amino acids necessary for the body's health. The tomatoes provide vitamin C and potassium, supporting heart health and immune function. Feta cheese adds calcium for bone health, while the spices contribute antioxidants, offering anti-inflammatory benefits. This dish is a wholesome choice for vegetarians seeking a hearty, low-carb meal to start their day.

6. Cauliflower and Cheese Breakfast Muffins

Prep time: 15 minutes
Cook time: 25 minutes
Serving size: 12 muffins

Ingredients:
- 2 cups riced cauliflower (about 1 medium head)
- 6 large eggs
- 1/2 cup almond flour
- 1 cup shredded cheddar cheese
- 1/4 cup finely chopped green onions
- 1/2 teaspoon garlic powder
- Salt and pepper to taste
- 1/4 teaspoon baking powder

Nutritional facts (per muffin):
- Calories: 120 kcal
- Carbohydrates: 3g

- Fiber: 1g

- Protein: 7g

- Fat: 9g

Preparation directions:

1. Preheat the oven to 375°F (190°C) and grease a muffin tin or line with paper liners.
2. Microwave the riced cauliflower in a covered bowl for 5 minutes, or until soft. Let it cool, then squeeze out excess water with a clean kitchen towel.
3. In a large bowl, whisk the eggs. Add the cooled cauliflower, almond flour, cheddar cheese, green onions, garlic powder, salt, pepper, and baking powder. Stir until well combined.
4. Evenly distribute the mixture into the prepared muffin tin cups, filling each about 3/4 full.
5. Bake in the preheated oven for 25 minutes, or until the tops are golden and a toothpick inserted into the center comes out clean.
6. Allow the muffins to cool for 5 minutes in the pan before transferring them to a wire rack to cool completely.

Health benefit:

Cauliflower and Cheese Breakfast Muffins are a nutritious and filling low-carb option, perfect for vegetarians looking for a quick breakfast. Cauliflower provides a high fiber content, which aids in digestion and helps to keep you feeling full longer. The eggs and cheese offer a good source of high-quality protein and calcium, supporting muscle health and bone density. Almond flour adds a dose of healthy fats and vitamin E, an important antioxidant. These muffins are a versatile and convenient breakfast choice, providing sustained energy without the spike in blood sugar levels.

7. Almond and Flaxseed Pancakes

Prep time: 10 minutes

Cook time: 15 minutes

Serving size: 4 servings (2 pancakes each)

Ingredients:

- 1 cup almond flour

- 1/4 cup ground flaxseed

- 2 large eggs

- 1/2 cup unsweetened almond milk

- 1 tablespoon melted coconut oil, plus more for cooking

- 1 teaspoon baking powder

- 1/2 teaspoon vanilla extract

- Pinch of salt

- Sweetener to taste (e.g., stevia or erythritol)

Nutritional facts (per serving):
- Calories: 230 kcal

- Carbohydrates: 8g

- Fiber: 5g

- Protein: 9g

- Fat: 19g

Preparation directions:

1. In a medium bowl, mix together almond flour, ground flaxseed, baking powder, and a pinch of salt.

2. In another bowl, whisk the eggs, almond milk, melted coconut oil, vanilla extract, and sweetener until well combined.

3. Pour the wet ingredients into the dry ingredients and stir until a batter forms. Let the batter sit for 5 minutes to thicken slightly.

4. Heat a non-stick skillet or griddle over medium heat and brush with a little coconut oil.

5. Pour 1/4 cup of batter for each pancake onto the skillet. Cook until bubbles form on the surface, then flip and cook until golden brown on the other side.

6. Serve warm with your choice of low-carb toppings, such as berries or sugar-free syrup.

Health benefit:

Almond and Flaxseed Pancakes offer a healthful, low-carb start to the day, rich in dietary fiber, healthy fats, and protein. The almond flour and flaxseed provide a substantial amount of omega-3 fatty acids, which are beneficial for heart health and cognitive function. These ingredients also contribute to the pancakes' high fiber content, promoting digestive health and helping to regulate blood sugar levels. The addition of eggs increases the protein content, making this meal satisfying and energizing, an ideal choice for vegetarians following a low-carb diet.

8. Coconut Yogurt with Nuts and Seeds

Prep time: 5 minutes
Serving size: 1 serving

Ingredients:

- 1 cup unsweetened coconut yogurt

- 1 tablespoon chia seeds

- 1 tablespoon flaxseed meal

- 2 tablespoons mixed nuts (almonds, walnuts, pecans), roughly chopped

- 1/4 teaspoon cinnamon

- Sweetener to taste (optional, e.g., stevia or erythritol)

Nutritional facts (per serving):

- Calories: 300 kcal

- Carbohydrates: 15g

- Fiber: 6g

- Protein: 8g

- Fat: 24g

Preparation directions:

1. In a serving bowl, combine the coconut yogurt with chia seeds, flaxseed meal, and cinnamon. Stir well to distribute the seeds evenly.
2. Add the sweetener, if using, and mix until well combined.
3. Top the yogurt mixture with the chopped mixed nuts.
4. Serve immediately, or refrigerate for 30 minutes to allow the chia seeds to swell and thicken the yogurt further.

Health benefit:

This Coconut Yogurt with Nuts and Seeds breakfast is a powerhouse of nutrition, offering a blend of healthy fats, proteins, and fibers that are essential for a balanced vegetarian diet. Coconut yogurt is a fantastic dairy-free alternative, providing probiotics that support digestive health. Chia seeds and flaxseed meal are excellent sources of omega-3 fatty acids, which contribute to heart health and help reduce inflammation. Nuts add not only a satisfying crunch but also supply additional protein and heart-healthy fats. This combination makes for a nutritious, filling breakfast that promotes sustained energy levels and overall well-being.

9. Bell Pepper and Kale Frittata

Prep time: 10 minutes

Cook time: 20 minutes

Serving size: 4 servings

Ingredients:

- 8 large eggs

- 1 cup chopped kale, stems removed

- 1 red bell pepper, diced

- 1/2 onion, diced

- 1/4 cup grated Parmesan cheese (optional for those who include dairy)

- 1 tablespoon olive oil

- Salt and pepper to taste

- 1/2 teaspoon garlic powder

Nutritional facts (per serving):

- Calories: 210 kcal

- Carbohydrates: 5g

- Fiber: 1g

- Protein: 14g

- Fat: 15g

Preparation directions:

1. Preheat the oven to 375°F (190°C).

2. Heat olive oil in an oven-safe skillet over medium heat. Add the diced bell pepper and onion, sautéing until softened, about 5 minutes.

3. Add the chopped kale and garlic powder to the skillet, and cook until the kale is wilted, about 2 minutes.

4. In a bowl, whisk together the eggs, salt, and pepper. Pour the egg mixture over the vegetables in the skillet.

5. Sprinkle the grated Parmesan cheese over the top, if using.

6. Transfer the skillet to the oven and bake for 15 minutes, or until the eggs are set and the top is lightly golden.

7. Remove from the oven, let cool slightly, and cut into wedges to serve.

Health benefit:

The Bell Pepper and Kale Frittata is a nutrient-dense breakfast option that provides a good balance of protein, healthy fats, and vegetables. Eggs are a complete protein source, supplying all essential amino acids needed for muscle repair and growth. Kale is rich in vitamins A, C, and K, as well as antioxidants and fiber, which support immune function, eye health, and digestion. Bell peppers add vitamin C and bioflavonoids, promoting healthy skin and reducing inflammation. This frittata is a satisfying, wholesome meal that supports a healthy, low-carb vegetarian lifestyle.

10. Pumpkin Spice Chia Pudding

Prep time: 10 minutes

Cook time: 0 minutes (requires at least 4 hours of refrigeration)

Serving size: 2 servings

Ingredients:

- 1/4 cup chia seeds

- 1 cup unsweetened almond milk

- 1/4 cup pumpkin puree (not pumpkin pie filling)

- 1/2 teaspoon pumpkin pie spice

- 1 tablespoon sugar-free maple syrup or sweetener of choice

- 1/4 teaspoon vanilla extract

Nutritional facts (per serving):

- Calories: 150 kcal

- Carbohydrates: 15g

- Fiber: 10g

- Protein: 4g

- Fat: 8g

Preparation directions:

1. In a bowl, combine the chia seeds, almond milk, pumpkin puree, pumpkin pie spice, sweetener, and vanilla extract. Mix well to ensure there are no clumps.

2. Cover the bowl and refrigerate for at least 4 hours, or overnight, until the pudding has thickened and the chia seeds have absorbed the liquid.

3. Stir the pudding before serving. If it's too thick, adjust the consistency by adding a little more almond milk.

4. Serve chilled, with an optional sprinkle of pumpkin pie spice or a few pecans on top for garnish.

Health benefit:

Pumpkin Spice Chia Pudding is a festive and healthful breakfast choice, especially in the fall. This pudding is rich in dietary fiber from the chia seeds, which promotes healthy digestion and helps to maintain stable blood sugar levels. Pumpkin puree is a great source of beta-carotene, which the body converts into vitamin A, supporting vision health and immune function. The addition of pumpkin pie spice not only provides seasonal flavor but also includes cinnamon, which has been shown to have anti-inflammatory properties. This breakfast is a delicious way to start the day with a meal that supports a low-carb vegetarian diet and overall health.

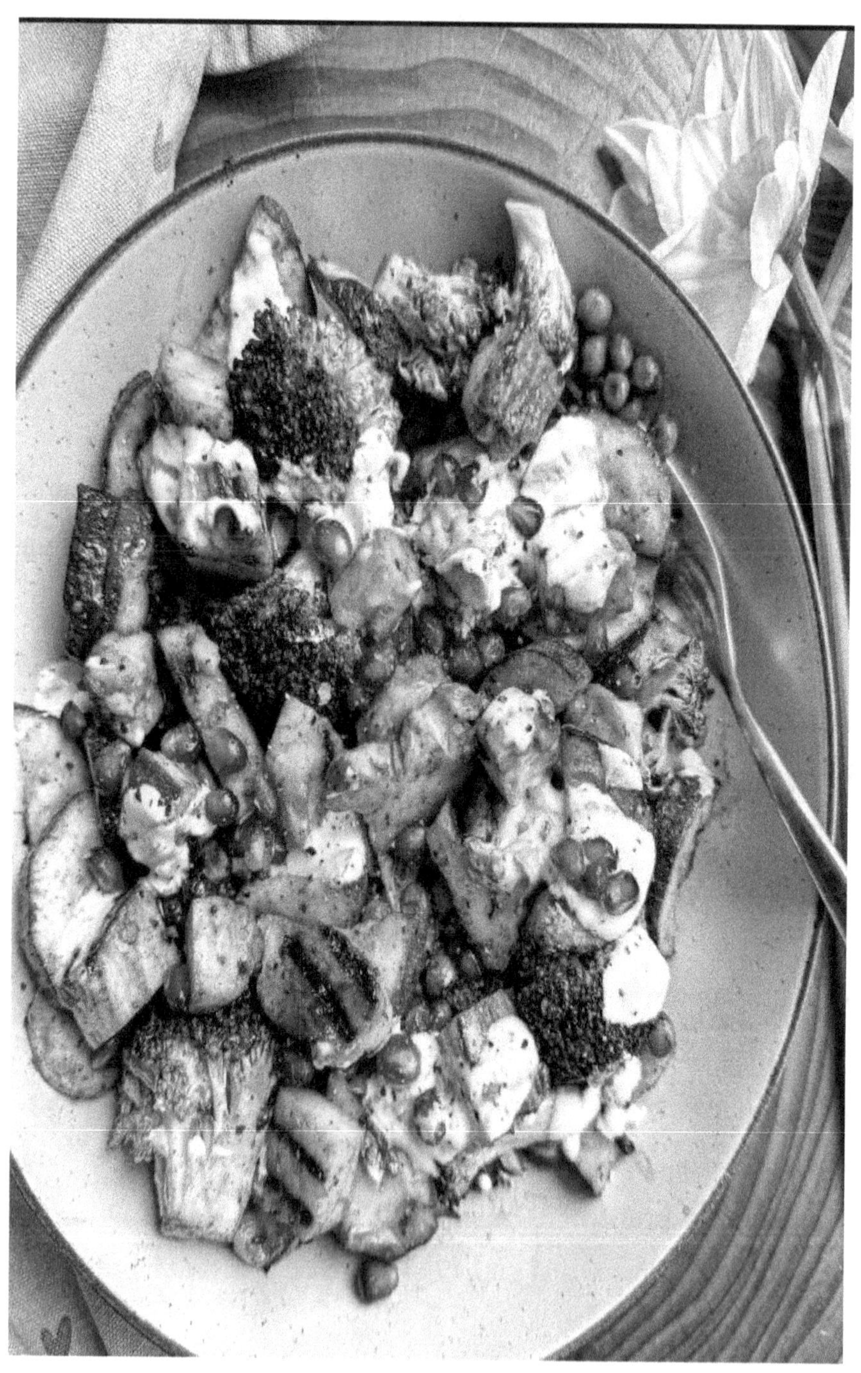

11. Zucchini Noodles with Avocado Pesto

Prep time: 10 minutes

Serving size: 2 servings

Ingredients:

- 2 medium zucchinis, spiralized

- 1 ripe avocado

- 1/2 cup fresh basil leaves

- 2 cloves garlic

- 2 tablespoons pine nuts

- 2 tablespoons lemon juice

- 1/4 cup extra-virgin olive oil

- Salt and pepper to taste

- Cherry tomatoes for garnish (optional)

Nutritional facts (per serving):

- Calories: 320 kcal

- Carbohydrates: 14g

- Fiber: 7g

- Protein: 4g

- Fat: 29g

Preparation directions:

1. Place the avocado, basil leaves, garlic, pine nuts, lemon juice, and half of the olive oil in a food processor. Blend until smooth, adding more olive oil as needed to reach a creamy consistency. Season with salt and pepper.
2. Spiralize the zucchinis to create noodles. If you prefer softer noodles, blanch them in boiling water for 1-2 minutes, then drain and pat dry.
3. In a large bowl, toss the zucchini noodles with the avocado pesto until evenly coatcd.
4. Serve immediately, garnished with cherry tomatoes if desired.

Health benefit:

Zucchini Noodles with Avocado Pesto is a heart-healthy, low-carb alternative to traditional pasta dishes, perfect for a nutritious lunch. Avocados are an excellent source of healthy monounsaturated fats, which can help lower bad cholesterol levels and reduce the risk of heart disease. Zucchini provides dietary fiber, promoting healthy digestion and aiding in weight management. This dish is also rich in vitamins C and K, along with antioxidants that support immune health and anti-inflammatory benefits, making it a satisfying and healthful choice for vegetarians.

12. Cauliflower Tabouleh

Prep time: 15 minutes

Serving size: 4 servings

Ingredients:

- 1 medium head of cauliflower, riced

- 1 cup fresh parsley, finely chopped

- 1/2 cup fresh mint, finely chopped

- 1/4 cup red onion, finely diced

- 1 cucumber, diced

- 2 medium tomatoes, deseeded and diced

- 3 tablespoons olive oil

- 2 tablespoons lemon juice

- Salt and pepper to taste

Nutritional facts (per serving):

- Calories: 130 kcal

- Carbohydrates: 12g

- Fiber: 4g

- Protein: 3g

- Fat: 9g

Preparation directions:

1. Rice the cauliflower by pulsing florets in a food processor until it resembles coarse grains. Avoid over-processing.
2. In a large mixing bowl, combine the riced cauliflower, chopped parsley, mint, red onion, cucumber, and tomatoes.
3. Drizzle with olive oil and lemon juice, then season with salt and pepper to taste. Toss well to combine all the ingredients.
4. Let the tabouleh sit for at least 10 minutes before serving to allow the flavors to meld.
5. Serve chilled or at room temperature.

Health benefit:

Cauliflower Tabouleh is a refreshing and nutritious alternative to traditional tabouleh, ideal for vegetarians seeking a low-carb option. Cauliflower serves as an excellent base, offering a rich source of vitamin C, vitamin K, and fiber, which support immune health, bone health, and digestive wellness. Parsley and mint add a burst of fresh flavor, along with a range of vitamins, minerals, and antioxidants that promote good health. This dish is also hydrating and can help to detoxify the body, making it a perfect light lunch or side dish.

13. Creamy Spinach Soup (Dairy-Free)

Prep time: 5 minutes

Cook time: 20 minutes

Serving size: 4 servings

Ingredients:

- 1 tablespoon olive oil

- 1 small onion, chopped

- 2 cloves garlic, minced

- 4 cups fresh spinach leaves

- 1 can (14 oz) coconut milk

- 2 cups vegetable broth

- Salt and pepper to taste

- Nutmeg for garnish (optional)

Nutritional facts (per serving):

- Calories: 220 kcal

- Carbohydrates: 7g

- Fiber: 1g

- Protein: 3g

- Fat: 21g

Preparation directions:

1. Heat the olive oil in a large pot over medium heat. Add the onion and garlic, sautéing until softened, about 5 minutes.
2. Add the spinach leaves to the pot, cooking until they wilt, about 2-3 minutes.
3. Pour in the coconut milk and vegetable broth, bringing the mixture to a simmer. Season with salt and pepper.
4. Simmer for 15 minutes, then blend the soup using an immersion blender or carefully transfer to a blender to process until smooth.
5. Serve hot, garnished with a sprinkle of nutmeg if desired.

Health benefit:

Creamy Spinach Soup offers a dairy-free, low-carb lunch option packed with nutrients essential for vegetarians. Spinach is a powerhouse of vitamins and minerals, including iron, magnesium, and vitamins A, C, and K, supporting blood health, bone health, and immune function. Coconut milk provides a source of medium-chain triglycerides (MCTs), which can aid in metabolism and energy production. This soup is comforting, satisfying, and beneficial for maintaining a healthy, balanced diet.

14. Greek Salad with Tofu Feta

Prep time: 15 minutes (plus marinating time for tofu)

Serving size: 4 servings

Ingredients:

- **For the Tofu Feta:**

  - 1 block (14 oz) extra-firm tofu, pressed and cubed

  - 1/4 cup apple cider vinegar

  - 1/4 cup lemon juice

  - 2 tablespoons olive oil

  - 1 teaspoon dried oregano

  - 1/2 teaspoon salt

  - 1/4 teaspoon black pepper

- **For the Salad:**

  - 4 cups mixed greens (romaine, spinach, arugula)

  - 1 cucumber, diced

  - 2 tomatoes, diced

  - 1/2 red onion, thinly sliced

  - 1/2 cup Kalamata olives

  - 1/4 cup chopped fresh parsley

Nutritional facts (per serving):

- Calories: 200 kcal

- Carbohydrates: 10g

- Fiber: 3g

- Protein: 12g

- Fat: 14g

Preparation directions:

1. To prepare the tofu feta, combine the cubed tofu with apple cider vinegar, lemon juice, olive oil, oregano, salt, and pepper in a bowl. Toss to coat evenly. Cover and refrigerate for at least 2 hours, preferably overnight, to marinate.

2. In a large salad bowl, combine the mixed greens, diced cucumber, diced tomatoes, sliced red onion, and Kalamata olives.

3. Add the marinated tofu feta to the salad and toss gently to combine.

4. Garnish with chopped fresh parsley before serving.

Health benefit:

Greek Salad with Tofu Feta is a refreshing and nutritious choice, offering a balance of protein, healthy fats, and a variety of vitamins and minerals. The tofu provides a high-quality plant-based protein source, making it an excellent option for vegetarians. Its preparation with vinegar and lemon juice not only adds flavor but also aids in digestion. The salad's vegetables contribute antioxidants, dietary fiber, and essential nutrients, supporting heart health, immune function, and overall well-being. This dish is a delightful way to enjoy a classic salad with a vegetarian twist.

15. Caprese Stuffed Avocado

Prep time: 10 minutes

Serving size: 2 servings

Ingredients:

- 2 ripe avocados, halved and pitted

- 1 cup cherry tomatoes, halved

- 1/2 cup mozzarella balls (use dairy-free if preferred), halved

- 1/4 cup fresh basil leaves, chopped

- 2 tablespoons balsamic glaze

- Salt and pepper to taste

- 1 tablespoon olive oil

Nutritional facts (per serving):

- Calories: 320 kcal

- Carbohydrates: 17g

- Fiber: 10g

- Protein: 8g

- Fat: 26g

Preparation directions:

1. Scoop out a little of the avocado flesh to create more space for the filling, leaving a border around the edges.
2. In a bowl, mix together the cherry tomatoes, mozzarella balls, and chopped basil. Season with salt and pepper.
3. Spoon the tomato and mozzarella mixture into the avocado halves.
4. Drizzle each stuffed avocado half with balsamic glaze and a little olive oil.
5. Serve immediately, enjoying the blend of creamy avocado with the classic caprese flavors.

Health benefit:

Caprese Stuffed Avocado combines healthy fats, proteins, and antioxidants in a simple yet flavorful dish. Avocados are a great source of monounsaturated fats, which are beneficial for heart health and can help lower cholesterol levels. The mozzarella provides calcium for bone health, while the tomatoes offer vitamin C and lycopene, an antioxidant known for its potential to reduce the risk of certain diseases. This dish is a visually appealing, nutrient-dense option that aligns well with a low-carb vegetarian lifestyle, providing satiety and health benefits in every bite.

16. Broccoli and Almond Salad

Prep time: 15 minutes

Serving size: 4 servings

Ingredients:

- 4 cups broccoli florets, raw or lightly steamed

- 1/2 cup sliced almonds, toasted

- 1/4 cup dried cranberries, sugar-free

- 1/4 cup red onion, finely chopped

For the dressing:

- 1/4 cup mayonnaise (use vegan mayo for a dairy-free option)

- 1 tablespoon apple cider vinegar

- 1 tablespoon lemon juice

- 1 tablespoon sugar-free sweetener (e.g., erythritol)

- Salt and pepper to taste

Nutritional facts (per serving):

- Calories: 220 kcal

- Carbohydrates: 12g

- Fiber: 4g

- Protein: 6g

- Fat: 18g

Preparation directions:

1. If you prefer your broccoli to be slightly tender, lightly steam the florets for about 2-3 minutes, then plunge into ice water to stop the cooking process. Drain well.
2. In a large bowl, combine the broccoli florets, sliced almonds, dried cranberries, and red onion.
3. In a small bowl, whisk together the mayonnaise, apple cider vinegar, lemon juice, sweetener, salt, and pepper to create the dressing.
4. Pour the dressing over the broccoli mixture and toss until evenly coated.
5. Refrigerate the salad for at least 30 minutes before serving to allow the flavors to meld together.

Health benefit:

Broccoli and Almond Salad is an excellent source of dietary fiber, vitamins, and minerals. Broccoli is rich in vitamin C, vitamin K, and folate, supporting immune function, bone health, and cell growth. Almonds add protein and healthy fats, including vitamin E, which acts as a powerful antioxidant to protect cells from oxidative damage. This salad is not only nourishing but also provides a crunchy texture and a blend of flavors that make it a satisfying low-carb lunch option for vegetarians.

17. Keto Eggplant Pizza Rounds

Prep time: 10 minutes

Cook time: 25 minutes

Serving size: 4 servings

Ingredients:

- 1 large eggplant, sliced into 1/2 inch rounds

- 1 cup low-carb marinara sauce

- 1 cup shredded mozzarella cheese (use dairy-free if preferred)

- 1/2 cup mini pepperoni slices (use vegetarian pepperoni or sliced olives for a vegetarian option)

- 1 tablespoon olive oil

- 1 teaspoon Italian seasoning

- Salt and pepper to taste

- Fresh basil leaves for garnish

Nutritional facts (per serving):

- Calories: 200 kcal

- Carbohydrates: 10g

- Fiber: 4g

- Protein: 12g

- Fat: 14g

Preparation directions:

1. Preheat the oven to 400°F (200°C). Line a baking sheet with parchment paper.
2. Arrange the eggplant rounds on the baking sheet. Brush both sides with olive oil and season with salt, pepper, and Italian seasoning.
3. Bake the eggplant rounds for 10 minutes, then flip and bake for another 5 minutes until slightly tender.
4. Remove from the oven and top each round with marinara sauce, shredded mozzarella, and vegetarian pepperoni or olives.
5. Return to the oven and bake for an additional 10 minutes, or until the cheese is melted and bubbly.
6. Garnish with fresh basil leaves before serving.

Health benefit:

Keto Eggplant Pizza Rounds offer a nutritious and low-carb alternative to traditional pizza, incorporating vegetables directly into the meal. Eggplant provides fiber, vitamins B1 and B6, and potassium, which support heart health and brain function. Using low-carb marinara sauce and topping with high-protein cheese (or dairy-free alternative) and vegetarian toppings enhances the dish's nutritional profile while keeping it aligned with vegetarian keto guidelines. This recipe is a fun and healthful way to satisfy pizza cravings without compromising dietary goals.

18. Cucumber Boat with Spicy Tofu Salad

Prep time: 15 minutes

Serving size: 2 servings

Ingredients:

- 1 large cucumber, halved lengthwise and seeded

- 1 cup firm tofu, drained and crumbled

- 1/4 cup red bell pepper, finely diced

- 1/4 cup carrot, shredded

- 2 tablespoons green onions, chopped

- 1 tablespoon cilantro, chopped

For the dressing:

- 2 tablespoons peanut butter (unsweetened)

- 1 tablespoon soy sauce (or tamari for gluten-free)

- 1 tablespoon lime juice

- 1 teaspoon sriracha (adjust to taste)

- 1 tablespoon water (or more for desired consistency)

- Crushed peanuts for garnish

Nutritional facts (per serving):

- Calories: 250 kcal

- Carbohydrates: 12g

- Fiber: 3g

- Protein: 14g

- Fat: 17g

Preparation directions:

1. In a medium bowl, combine the crumbled tofu, red bell pepper, carrot, green onions, and cilantro.

2. In a small bowl, whisk together the peanut butter, soy sauce, lime juice, sriracha, and water until smooth. Adjust the consistency with more water if needed.

3. Pour the dressing over the tofu mixture and toss until well coated.

4. Spoon the spicy tofu salad into the cucumber halves, creating "boats."

5. Garnish with crushed peanuts before serving.

Health benefit:

The Cucumber Boat with Spicy Tofu Salad is a refreshing and protein-rich lunch option, perfect for a low-carb vegetarian diet. Tofu is an excellent source of plant-based protein and contains all nine essential amino acids, making it a complete protein source for vegetarians. The vegetables add crunch, fiber, and essential nutrients, while the spicy peanut dressing provides healthy fats and a flavorful kick. This dish is hydrating, satisfying, and packed with nutrients that support muscle health, digestion, and overall well-being.

19. Asparagus and Artichoke Heart Salad

Prep time: 15 minutes

Cook time: 5 minutes

Serving size: 4 servings

Ingredients:

- 1 pound asparagus, trimmed and cut into 2-inch pieces

- 1 can (14 oz) artichoke hearts, drained and quartered

- 1/4 cup red onion, thinly sliced

- 1/4 cup cherry tomatoes, halved

- 1/4 cup kalamata olives, halved

- 2 tablespoons olive oil

- 1 tablespoon lemon juice

- 1 teaspoon Dijon mustard

- Salt and pepper to taste

- Shaved Parmesan cheese (optional, use dairy-free if preferred)

Nutritional facts (per serving):

- Calories: 150 kcal

- Carbohydrates: 14g

- Fiber: 7g

- Protein: 5g

- Fat: 9g

Preparation directions:

1. Blanch the asparagus in boiling water for 2-3 minutes until bright green and tender-crisp. Immediately transfer to an ice bath to stop the cooking process. Drain well.

2. In a large salad bowl, combine the blanched asparagus, artichoke hearts, red onion, cherry tomatoes, and kalamata olives.

3. In a small bowl, whisk together the olive oil, lemon juice, Dijon mustard, salt, and pepper to create the dressing.

4. Pour the dressing over the salad and toss gently to coat evenly.

5. Serve the salad garnished with shaved Parmesan cheese, if using.

Health benefit:

Asparagus and Artichoke Heart Salad is a light, nutrient-dense dish that is perfect for a low-carb lunch. Asparagus is a great source of fiber, folate, and vitamins A, C, and K, supporting digestive health, cell growth, and immune function. Artichokes are rich in antioxidants and fiber, aiding in digestion and heart health. The addition of healthy fats from olive oil and the optional Parmesan cheese provides satiety and flavor, making this salad a well-rounded, nutritious option for vegetarians.

20. Roasted Red Pepper and Goat Cheese Zucchini Rolls

Prep time: 20 minutes

Serving size: 2 servings

Ingredients:

- 2 large zucchinis, thinly sliced lengthwise

- 1 cup roasted red peppers, cut into strips

- 4 ounces goat cheese, softened (use dairy-free cheese if preferred)

- 1/4 cup basil leaves, chopped

- Salt and pepper to taste

- 1 tablespoon olive oil

- Balsamic glaze for drizzling (optional)

Nutritional facts (per serving):

- Calories: 250 kcal

- Carbohydrates: 8g

- Fiber: 2g

- Protein: 11g

- Fat: 20g

Preparation directions:

1. Use a vegetable peeler or mandoline to slice the zucchinis into thin, long strips.
2. Lay out the zucchini strips on a flat surface and season lightly with salt and pepper.
3. Spread a thin layer of goat cheese on each zucchini strip.
4. Place a few strips of roasted red pepper and a sprinkle of chopped basil on one end of each zucchini strip.
5. Carefully roll up the zucchini strips, starting from the end with the fillings.
6. Arrange the zucchini rolls on a serving platter. Drizzle with olive oil and balsamic glaze if desired.

Health benefit:

Roasted Red Pepper and Goat Cheese Zucchini Rolls are a delightful, low-carb lunch option that provides a good balance of vegetables, protein, and healthy fats. Zucchini is low in calories but high in antioxidants and vitamin C, supporting skin health and immune function. Goat cheese offers a creamy texture and a good source of protein and calcium. Roasted red peppers add sweetness and are high in vitamins C and A, promoting eye health and antioxidant protection. This dish is visually appealing, easy to make, and packed with flavors and nutrients beneficial for a healthy vegetarian diet.

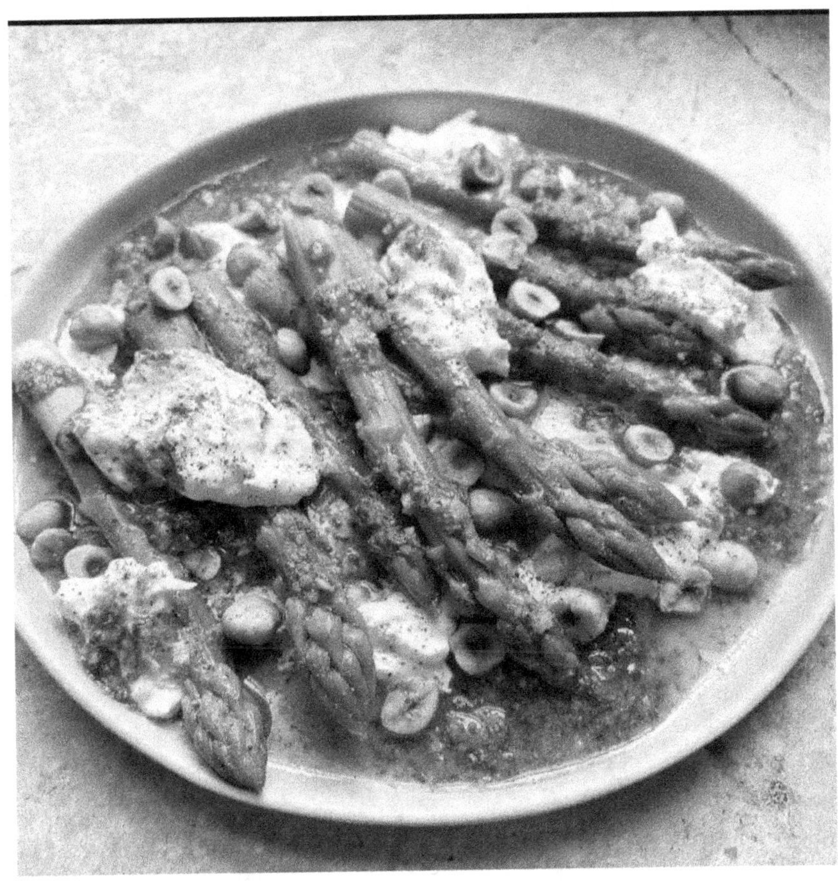

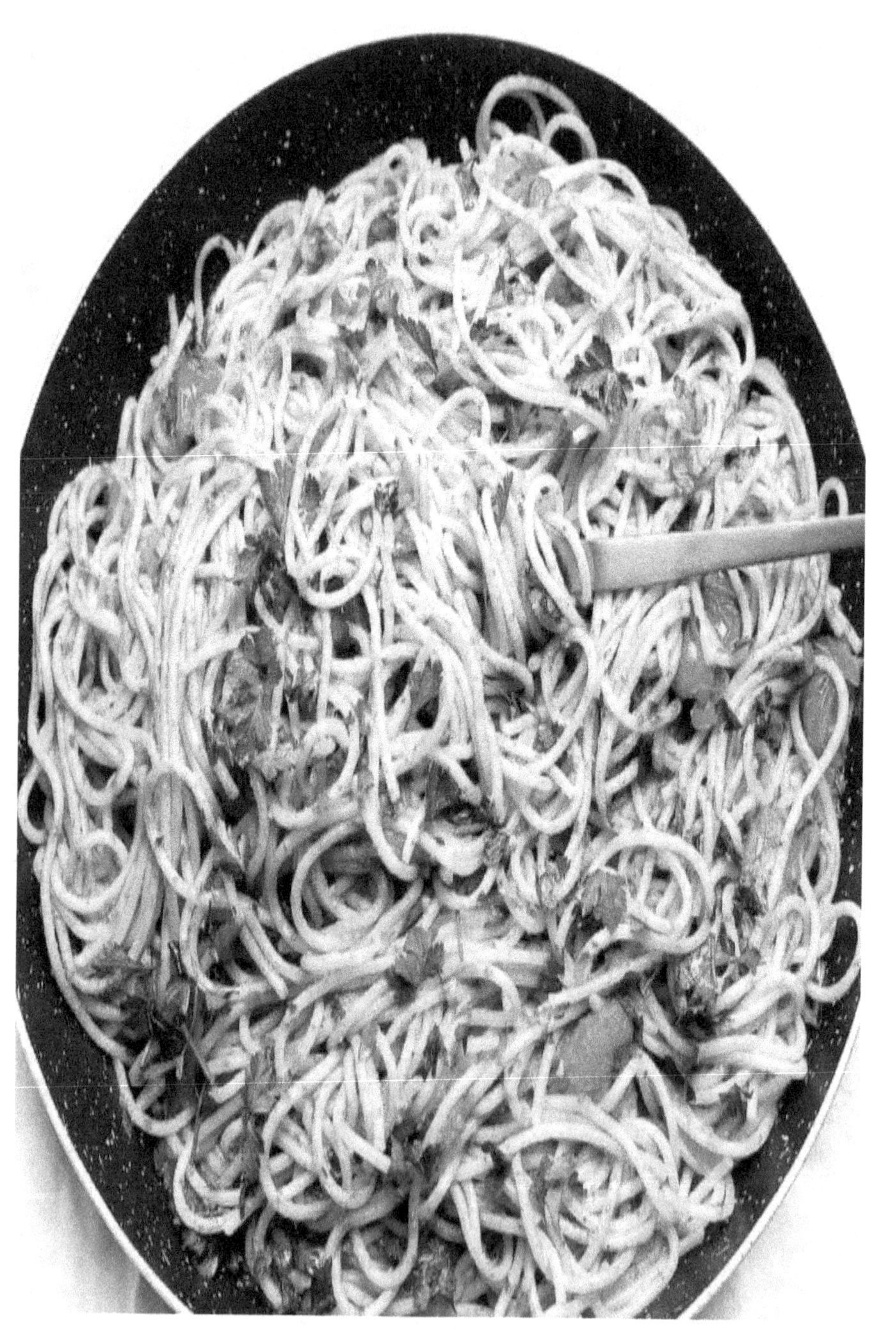

21. Mushroom Stroganoff (Zucchini Noodles)

Prep time: 15 minutes
Cook time: 20 minutes
Serving size: 4 servings

Ingredients:

- 4 large zucchinis, spiralized

- 2 tablespoons olive oil

- 1 pound mushrooms, sliced (mix of button, cremini, and/or portobello)

- 1 small onion, finely chopped

- 2 cloves garlic, minced

- 1 cup vegetable broth

- 1/2 cup sour cream (use a vegan alternative for dairy-free)

- 2 tablespoons soy sauce or tamari

- 1 tablespoon Dijon mustard

- Salt and pepper to taste

- Fresh parsley, chopped, for garnish

Nutritional facts (per serving):

- Calories: 180 kcal

- Carbohydrates: 12g

- Fiber: 3g

- Protein: 6g

- Fat: 12g

Preparation directions:

1. Heat one tablespoon of olive oil in a large skillet over medium heat. Add the spiralized zucchini noodles and sauté for 2-3 minutes until just tender. Remove from the skillet and set aside.

2. In the same skillet, add the remaining tablespoon of olive oil, mushrooms, onion, and garlic. Cook over medium heat until the mushrooms are browned and the onions are soft, about 8-10 minutes.

3. Add the vegetable broth, soy sauce, and Dijon mustard to the skillet. Stir to combine and bring to a simmer. Reduce heat and simmer for 5 minutes.

4. Stir in the sour cream and season with salt and pepper to taste. Continue to cook on low heat until the sauce is heated through, about 2 minutes.

5. Serve the mushroom stroganoff over the zucchini noodles, garnished with chopped parsley.

Health benefit:

Mushroom Stroganoff with Zucchini Noodles offers a comforting and nutritious dinner option, rich in vitamins and minerals. Mushrooms provide a meaty texture and are a good source of B vitamins, selenium, potassium, and antioxidants, supporting immune function and reducing inflammation. Zucchini noodles are a low-carb, high-fiber alternative to traditional pasta, aiding in digestion and weight management. This dish is a creamy, satisfying meal that combines the health benefits of vegetables with the indulgence of stroganoff, making it an excellent choice for a low-carb vegetarian dinner.

22. Cauliflower Steak with Chimichurri Sauce

Prep time: 10 minutes

Cook time: 25 minutes

Serving size: 4 servings

Ingredients:

- 2 large heads of cauliflower

- 3 tablespoons olive oil

- Salt and pepper to taste

- For the Chimichurri Sauce:

- 1 cup fresh parsley, finely chopped

- 1/4 cup fresh cilantro, finely chopped

- 1/2 cup olive oil

- 1/4 cup red wine vinegar

- 3 cloves garlic, minced

- 1 teaspoon red pepper flakes

- Salt and pepper to taste

Nutritional facts (per serving):

- Calories: 300 kcal

- Carbohydrates: 8g

- Fiber: 3g

- Protein: 4g

- Fat: 28g

Preparation directions:

1. Preheat the oven to 400°F (200°C). Line a baking sheet with parchment paper.

2. Slice the cauliflower heads into 1-inch thick steaks, being careful to keep the florets attached to the core. You should get about 2 steaks per head.

3. Brush both sides of each cauliflower steak with olive oil and season with salt and pepper.

4. Place the cauliflower steaks on the prepared baking sheet and roast in the oven for about 25 minutes, flipping halfway through, until tender and golden.

5. While the cauliflower is roasting, prepare the chimichurri sauce by combining parsley, cilantro, olive oil, red wine vinegar, garlic, red pepper flakes, salt, and pepper in a bowl. Stir until well mixed.

6. Serve the roasted cauliflower steaks drizzled with the chimichurri sauce.

Health benefit:

Cauliflower Steak with Chimichurri Sauce is a hearty, flavorful dish that provides a wealth of nutritional benefits. Cauliflower is an excellent source of vitamins C and K, folate, and fiber, promoting heart health and providing anti-inflammatory properties. The chimichurri sauce, made with herbs, olive oil, and vinegar, offers antioxidants and healthy fats, which can help to reduce the risk of chronic diseases and improve overall heart health. This dish is a fantastic way to enjoy a vegetarian steak alternative that's both satisfying and packed with essential nutrients.

23. Spaghetti Squash with Creamy Mushroom Sauce

Prep time: 10 minutes

Cook time: 45 minutes

Serving size: 4 servings

Ingredients:

- 1 large spaghetti squash, halved lengthwise and seeds removed
- 2 tablespoons olive oil, divided
- Salt and pepper to taste
- 1 pound mushrooms, sliced (a mix of cremini, portobello, and shiitake)
- 2 cloves garlic, minced
- 1 cup vegetable broth
- 1/2 cup coconut cream
- 1 teaspoon thyme, fresh or dried
- 2 tablespoons nutritional yeast (optional for a cheesy flavor)
- Fresh parsley, chopped, for garnish

Nutritional facts (per serving):

- Calories: 220 kcal
- Carbohydrates: 18g
- Fiber: 4g

- Protein: 4g

- Fat: 16g

Preparation directions:

1. Preheat the oven to 400°F (200°C). Brush the cut sides of the spaghetti squash with 1 tablespoon of olive oil and season with salt and pepper.

2. Place the squash cut side down on a baking sheet and roast for 35-40 minutes, or until tender and the flesh easily shreds with a fork.

3. While the squash is roasting, heat the remaining olive oil in a large skillet over medium heat. Add the mushrooms and garlic, sautéing until the mushrooms are golden and tender, about 8 minutes.

4. Pour in the vegetable broth, coconut cream, and thyme. Bring to a simmer and cook until the sauce thickens slightly, about 10 minutes. Stir in the nutritional yeast if using, and season with salt and pepper to taste.

5. Once the spaghetti squash is cooked, use a fork to scrape the inside flesh into strands, creating "spaghetti."

6. Divide the spaghetti squash among plates and top with the creamy mushroom sauce. Garnish with fresh parsley before serving.

Health benefit:

Spaghetti Squash with Creamy Mushroom Sauce is a comforting and nutritious low-carb dinner option. Spaghetti squash is a great source of vitamins A, C, and B vitamins, as well as fiber, which supports digestive health and can help regulate blood sugar levels. Mushrooms provide selenium, potassium, and B vitamins, which boost the immune system and support brain health. The coconut cream adds a dairy-free richness to the sauce, offering healthy fats and making this dish both satisfying and suitable for a variety of dietary preferences. This meal is a wonderful way to enjoy a "pasta-like" experience without the added carbohydrates.

24. Baked Tofu with Peanut Sauce and Stir-Fry Veggies

Prep time: 20 minutes (plus marinating time)

Cook time: 30 minutes

Serving size: 4 servings

Ingredients:

- **For the Baked Tofu:**

  - 1 block (14 oz) extra-firm tofu, pressed and cubed

  - 2 tablespoons soy sauce

  - 1 tablespoon sesame oil

  - 1 tablespoon maple syrup

- For the Peanut Sauce:

  - 1/4 cup natural peanut butter

  - 2 tablespoons soy sauce

  - 1 tablespoon lime juice

  - 1 tablespoon maple syrup

  - 1 teaspoon grated ginger

  - Water, as needed to thin the sauce

- For the Stir-Fry Veggies:

  - 2 tablespoons vegetable oil

  - 4 cups mixed vegetables (bell peppers, broccoli, carrots, snap peas)

  - Salt and pepper to taste

Nutritional facts (per serving):

- Calories: 350 kcal

- Carbohydrates: 24g

- Fiber: 4g

- Protein: 18g

- Fat: 22g

Preparation directions:

1. Marinate the tofu cubes in a mixture of soy sauce, sesame oil, and maple syrup for at least 30 minutes, preferably longer.

2. Preheat the oven to 400°F (200°C). Arrange the marinated tofu on a baking sheet lined with parchment paper. Bake for 25-30 minutes, until crispy and golden.

3. For the peanut sauce, whisk together peanut butter, soy sauce, lime juice, maple syrup, and ginger in a bowl. Gradually add water until you achieve a smooth, pourable consistency.

4. Heat the vegetable oil in a large skillet or wok over medium-high heat. Add the mixed vegetables and stir-fry until tender-crisp, about 5-7 minutes. Season with salt and pepper.

5. Serve the baked tofu over the stir-fried vegetables and drizzle with peanut sauce.

Health benefit:

Baked Tofu with Peanut Sauce and Stir-Fry Veggies is a balanced meal that provides a high protein content from tofu, making it an excellent choice for vegetarians. Tofu is a complete protein source, containing all nine essential amino acids necessary for the body. The vegetables add a variety of vitamins, minerals, and fiber, promoting overall health and supporting digestion. Peanut sauce not only enhances the dish with its rich, savory flavor but also contributes healthy fats and additional protein. This meal is an enjoyable way to ensure a nutritious end to the day, packed with beneficial ingredients for a vegetarian diet.

25. Grilled Halloumi with Mediterranean Vegetables

Prep time: 15 minutes

Cook time: 20 minutes

Serving size: 4 servings

Ingredients:

- 8 oz halloumi cheese, sliced

- 2 zucchinis, sliced lengthwise

- 2 red bell peppers, deseeded and cut into large pieces

- 1 eggplant, sliced into rounds

- 2 tablespoons olive oil

- 1 teaspoon dried oregano

- Salt and pepper to taste

- Fresh basil leaves, for garnish

- Balsamic glaze, for drizzling (optional)

Nutritional facts (per serving):

- Calories: 320 kcal

- Carbohydrates: 15g

- Fiber: 5g

- Protein: 15g

- Fat: 22g

Preparation directions:

1. Preheat the grill to medium-high heat.

2. Brush the halloumi, zucchinis, bell peppers, and eggplant slices with olive oil. Season with dried oregano, salt, and pepper.

3. Grill the vegetables for about 3-4 minutes on each side, until they are tender and have grill marks.

4. Grill the halloumi slices for 2-3 minutes on each side, until they are golden and slightly crispy.

5. Arrange the grilled vegetables and halloumi on a serving platter. Garnish with fresh basil leaves and drizzle with balsamic glaze if desired.

6. Serve immediately, enjoying the combination of flavors.

Health benefit:

Grilled Halloumi with Mediterranean Vegetables is a nutrient-rich, flavorful dish that offers a variety of health benefits. Halloumi cheese provides a good source of protein and calcium, important for bone health. The vegetables contribute a wealth of vitamins, minerals, and antioxidants, with zucchini offering vitamin C, bell peppers rich in vitamins A and C, and eggplant providing fiber and anthocyanins. Grilling vegetables preserves their nutritional content while enhancing their natural flavors. This dish is an excellent way to enjoy a balanced, vegetarian meal that supports overall health.

26. Vegan Alfredo with Shirataki Noodles

Prep time: 10 minutes
Cook time: 15 minutes
Serving size: 4 servings

Ingredients:

- 2 (8 oz) packages shirataki noodles, rinsed and drained

- 1 cup raw cashews, soaked for 4 hours and drained

- 1 cup vegetable broth

- 2 cloves garlic

- 2 tablespoons nutritional yeast

- 1 tablespoon lemon juice

- Salt and pepper to taste

- 1 tablespoon olive oil

- 1/2 cup chopped parsley, for garnish

Nutritional facts (per serving):

- Calories: 240 kcal

- Carbohydrates: 10g

- Fiber: 3g

- Protein: 8g

- Fat: 19g

Preparation directions:

1. Prepare the shirataki noodles according to the package instructions, typically rinsed under cold water and boiled for 2-3 minutes. Drain and set aside.

2. In a blender, combine the soaked cashews, vegetable broth, garlic, nutritional yeast, lemon juice, salt, and pepper. Blend until the mixture is smooth and creamy, adjusting the seasoning as needed.

3. Heat the olive oil in a large skillet over medium heat. Add the prepared shirataki noodles and sauté for 2-3 minutes to remove any excess moisture.

4. Reduce the heat to low and pour the vegan Alfredo sauce over the noodles. Stir well to coat the noodles evenly and heat through for another 2-3 minutes.

5. Serve the noodles garnished with chopped parsley.

Health benefit:

Vegan Alfredo with Shirataki Noodles is a low-carb, high-nutrient dinner option that satisfies cravings for creamy pasta without the heavy carbs. Shirataki noodles are made from the konjac plant, providing a fiber-rich, calorie-light alternative to traditional pasta. Cashews offer healthy fats, protein, and magnesium, which is beneficial for heart health and bone strength. Nutritional yeast adds a cheesy flavor along with B-vitamins, particularly B12, which is important for vegetarians. This dish is a great way to enjoy a classic comfort food in a healthier, plant-based form.

27. Vegetable Korma (Cauliflower Rice)

Prep time: 15 minutes
Cook time: 20 minutes
Serving size: 4 servings

Ingredients:

- 1 head of cauliflower, riced

- 2 tablespoons coconut oil

- 1 onion, diced

- 2 cloves garlic, minced

- 1 inch ginger, grated

- 2 carrots, diced

- 1 bell pepper, diced

- 1 cup green beans, chopped

- 1 cup peas (fresh or frozen)

- 1 can (14 oz) coconut milk

- 2 tablespoons curry powder

- 1 teaspoon turmeric

- Salt and pepper to taste

- Fresh cilantro, for garnish

Nutritional facts (per serving):

- Calories: 250 kcal

- Carbohydrates: 18g

- Fiber: 6g

- Protein: 5g

- Fat: 18g

Preparation directions:

1. Heat the coconut oil in a large skillet over medium heat. Add the onion, garlic, and ginger, sautéing until the onion is translucent, about 5 minutes.

2. Add the carrots, bell pepper, green beans, and peas to the skillet. Cook for another 5-7 minutes, until the vegetables are tender but still crisp.

3. Stir in the curry powder and turmeric, cooking for 1 minute until fragrant.

4. Pour in the coconut milk and bring the mixture to a simmer. Reduce heat and cook for 10 minutes, allowing the flavors to meld together.

5. Meanwhile, prepare the cauliflower rice by pulsing cauliflower florets in a food processor until it resembles rice. Briefly sauté in a separate pan with a little oil, salt, and pepper for 5-7 minutes.

6. Serve the vegetable korma over the cauliflower rice, garnished with fresh cilantro.

Health benefit:

Vegetable Korma served with Cauliflower Rice is a vibrant, nutrient-dense meal that's perfect for a low-carb vegetarian diet. The variety of vegetables used in the korma provides a wide range of vitamins, minerals, and fiber, supporting overall health and digestion. Cauliflower rice is a low-calorie, high-fiber alternative to traditional rice, aiding in weight management and blood sugar control. Coconut milk adds a creamy texture and healthy fats, particularly medium-chain triglycerides (MCTs), which can support metabolism. This dish is a flavorful way to enjoy a range of vegetables, making it a wholesome and satisfying dinner option.

28. Stuffed Bell Peppers (Quinoa and Vegetables)

Prep time: 20 minutes

Cook time: 30 minutes

Serving size: 4 servings

Ingredients:

- 4 large bell peppers, tops removed and seeded
- 1 cup quinoa, cooked according to package instructions
- 1 tablespoon olive oil
- 1 small onion, diced
- 2 cloves garlic, minced
- 1 zucchini, diced
- 1 cup spinach, chopped
- 1/2 cup cherry tomatoes, halved
- 1/4 cup fresh basil, chopped
- 1/2 cup feta cheese, crumbled (use vegan feta for a dairy-free option)
- Salt and pepper to taste

Nutritional facts (per serving):

- Calories: 280 kcal
- Carbohydrates: 38g

- Fiber: 6g

- Protein: 10g

- Fat: 10g

Preparation directions:

1. Preheat the oven to 375°F (190°C). Place the hollowed-out bell peppers in a baking dish.

2. Heat the olive oil in a large skillet over medium heat. Add the onion and garlic, sautéing until softened, about 5 minutes.

3. Add the zucchini and cook for an additional 5 minutes until just tender.

4. Stir in the cooked quinoa, spinach, cherry tomatoes, and basil. Cook until the spinach is wilted, about 2 minutes. Remove from heat and let cool slightly.

5. Mix in the crumbled feta cheese and season the filling with salt and pepper.

6. Spoon the filling into each bell pepper cavity, pressing down lightly to pack the filling.

7. Cover the baking dish with aluminum foil and bake in the preheated oven for about 25-30 minutes, until the peppers are tender and the filling is heated through.

8. Serve the stuffed peppers warm, optionally garnished with more fresh basil or a drizzle of olive oil.

Health benefit:

Stuffed Bell Peppers with Quinoa and Vegetables offer a balanced meal packed with nutrients. Quinoa is a complete protein source, containing all nine essential amino acids, making it an excellent choice for vegetarians. Bell peppers are high in vitamin C and antioxidants, supporting immune health and reducing inflammation. The inclusion of a variety of vegetables adds dietary fiber, vitamins, and minerals, promoting digestive health and providing a wide range of nutrients. Feta cheese (or its vegan alternative) adds calcium and flavor, making this dish not only nutritious but also delicious and satisfying.

29. Paneer Tikka Skewers

Prep time: 15 minutes (plus marinating time)
Cook time: 15 minutes
Serving size: 4 servings

Ingredients:

- 14 oz paneer cheese, cut into cubes

- 1 cup Greek yogurt (use vegan yogurt for dairy-free)

- 2 tablespoons tandoori masala

- 1 teaspoon turmeric

- 1 teaspoon garam masala

- 1 tablespoon lemon juice

- Salt to taste

- 1 bell pepper, cut into pieces

- 1 onion, cut into pieces

- 1 zucchini, cut into pieces

- Olive oil, for brushing

Nutritional facts (per serving):

- Calories: 350 kcal

- Carbohydrates: 10g

- Fiber: 2g

- Protein: 18g

- Fat: 26g

Preparation directions:

1. In a large bowl, mix the Greek yogurt, tandoori masala, turmeric, garam masala, lemon juice, and salt to create the marinade.

2. Add the paneer cubes to the marinade, ensuring each piece is well coated. Cover and refrigerate for at least 1 hour, preferably longer.

3. Preheat the grill to medium-high heat. Thread the marinated paneer, bell pepper, onion, and zucchini pieces onto skewers.

4. Brush the grill with olive oil and place the skewers on the grill. Cook, turning occasionally, for about 12-15 minutes, or until the paneer is golden brown and the vegetables are tender.

5. Serve the skewers hot, garnished with lemon wedges and fresh cilantro if desired.

Health benefit:

Paneer Tikka Skewers are a high-protein, flavorful dish that brings a wealth of nutritional benefits. Paneer cheese is a great source of calcium and protein, which are essential for bone health and muscle maintenance. The spices used in the marinade, such as turmeric and garam masala, offer anti-inflammatory properties and antioxidants, supporting overall health. The vegetables add fiber, vitamins, and minerals, making this dish not only delicious but also balanced and nutritious. Grilling the skewers enhances the flavors while keeping the meal light and healthful.

30. Moroccan Tagine with Turnip and Zucchini

Prep time: 20 minutes
Cook time: 40 minutes
Serving size: 4 servings

Ingredients:

- 2 tablespoons olive oil

- 1 onion, chopped

- 2 cloves garlic, minced

- 1 teaspoon ground cumin

- 1 teaspoon ground coriander

- 1/2 teaspoon cinnamon

- 1/4 teaspoon cayenne pepper (adjust to taste)

- 1 large turnip, peeled and cubed

- 2 zucchinis, cubed

- 1 can (14 oz) diced tomatoes

- 1 can (14 oz) chickpeas, rinsed and drained

- 2 cups vegetable broth

- Salt and pepper to taste

- Fresh cilantro, for garnish

- Cooked couscous or cauliflower rice, for serving

Nutritional facts (per serving, without couscous/cauliflower rice):

- Calories: 250 kcal
- Carbohydrates: 35g
- Fiber: 9g
- Protein: 8g
- Fat: 10g

Preparation directions:

1. Heat the olive oil in a large pot or tagine over medium heat. Add the onion and garlic, cooking until softened, about 5 minutes.
2. Stir in the cumin, coriander, cinnamon, and cayenne pepper, cooking for another minute until fragrant.
3. Add the turnip and zucchini, tossing to coat with the spices.
4. Pour in the diced tomatoes, chickpeas, and vegetable broth. Bring to a simmer, then reduce the heat, cover, and cook for 30-35 minutes, until the vegetables are tender.
5. Season with salt and pepper to taste. Serve the tagine hot, garnished with fresh cilantro, over cooked couscous or cauliflower rice.

Health benefit:

Moroccan Tagine with Turnip and Zucchini is a hearty, plant-based meal filled with spices that not only contribute rich flavors but also offer health benefits, including anti-inflammatory properties and antioxidants. The variety of vegetables and chickpeas in this dish provides a high fiber content, supporting digestive health and aiding in blood sugar regulation. Turnips are a good source of vitamin C, potassium, and calcium, while zucchinis offer vitamins A and C, supporting immune function and skin health. This dish is a flavorful way to enjoy a diverse range of nutrients in a comforting, one-pot meal.

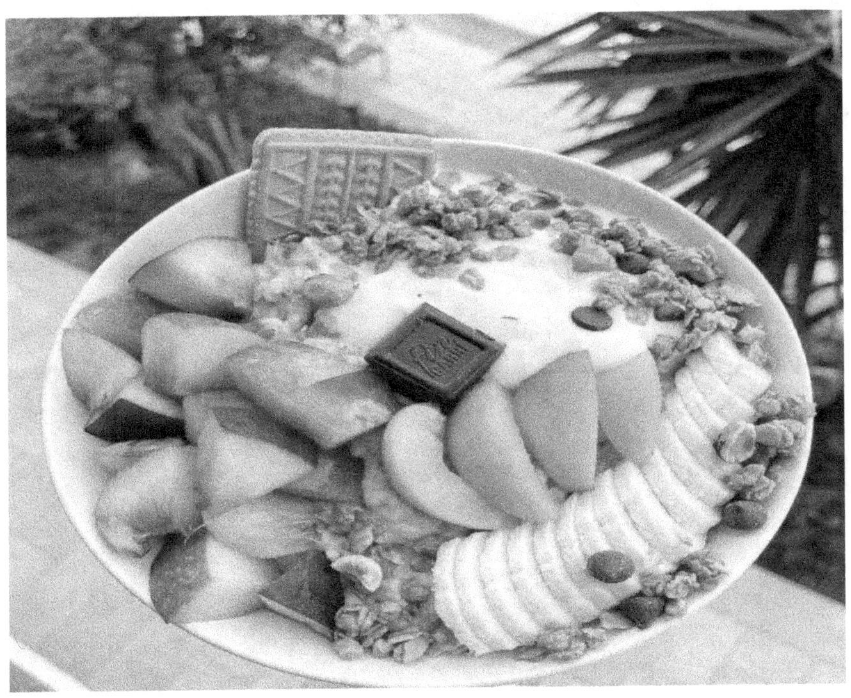

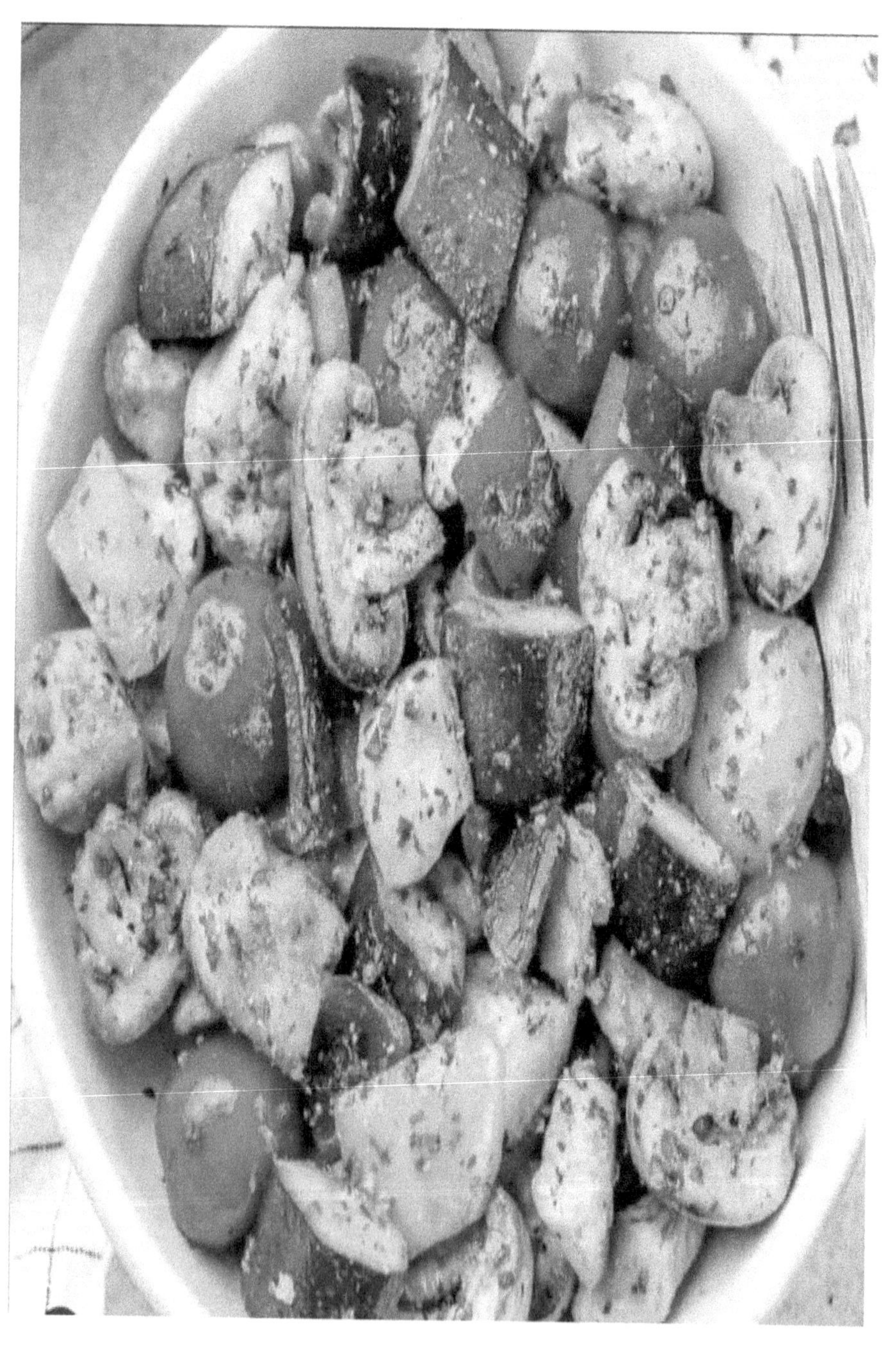

31. Avocado and Walnut Salad

Prep time: 10 minutes

Serving size: 4 servings

Ingredients:

- 2 ripe avocados, peeled, pitted, and diced

- 1/2 cup walnuts, toasted and roughly chopped

- 2 cups mixed salad greens (e.g., arugula, spinach, and romaine)

- 1/4 cup red onion, thinly sliced

- **For the dressing:**

  - 3 tablespoons extra virgin olive oil

  - 1 tablespoon balsamic vinegar

  - 1 teaspoon Dijon mustard

  - Salt and pepper to taste

Nutritional facts (per serving):

- Calories: 280 kcal

- Carbohydrates: 12g

- Fiber: 7g

- Protein: 4g

- Fat: 26g

Preparation directions:

1. In a large salad bowl, combine the diced avocados, toasted walnuts, mixed salad greens, and red onion.
2. In a small bowl, whisk together the olive oil, balsamic vinegar, Dijon mustard, salt, and pepper to create the dressing.
3. Drizzle the dressing over the salad and gently toss to coat all the ingredients evenly.
4. Serve immediately, offering a fresh and flavorful low-carb side or snack.

Health benefit:

Avocado and Walnut Salad is a nutrient-dense option that provides healthy fats, fiber, and a variety of vitamins and minerals. Avocados are rich in monounsaturated fats, which are beneficial for heart health, and are a great source of potassium and vitamin E. Walnuts add omega-3 fatty acids, known for their anti-inflammatory properties and brain health benefits. The mixed greens contribute antioxidants and vitamins A, C, and K, supporting overall health. This salad is a wholesome choice for a quick snack or side, promoting satiety and nourishment.

32. Keto Garlic Bread Sticks (Cauliflower Base)

Prep time: 15 minutes

Cook time: 25 minutes

Serving size: 8 breadsticks

Ingredients:

- 1 medium head of cauliflower, riced and cooked

- 1 egg, beaten

- 1/2 cup shredded mozzarella cheese (use dairy-free cheese for vegan option)

- 1/4 cup Parmesan cheese, grated (use nutritional yeast for vegan option)

- 2 cloves garlic, minced

- 1/2 teaspoon dried oregano

- 1/2 teaspoon dried basil

- Salt and pepper to taste

- Olive oil, for brushing

- Fresh parsley, chopped, for garnish

Nutritional facts (per breadstick):

- Calories: 70 kcal

- Carbohydrates: 4g

- Fiber: 2g

- Protein: 5g

- Fat: 4g

Preparation directions:

1. Preheat the oven to 400°F (200°C) and line a baking sheet with parchment paper.
2. Squeeze excess moisture from the cooked cauliflower rice using a clean kitchen towel.
3. In a bowl, combine the drained cauliflower rice, egg, mozzarella, Parmesan (or nutritional yeast), garlic, oregano, basil, salt, and pepper.
4. Spread the mixture onto the prepared baking sheet, forming a rectangle about 1/4 inch thick.
5. Bake in the preheated oven for 18-20 minutes, until golden and firm.
6. Brush the top with olive oil and broil for an additional 2-3 minutes to get a crispy surface.
7. Cut into breadsticks, garnish with fresh parsley, and serve warm.

Health benefit:

Keto Garlic Bread Sticks with a Cauliflower Base are an innovative, low-carb alternative to traditional garlic bread.

Cauliflower provides a good source of vitamin C, potassium, and fiber, aiding in digestion and contributing to overall health. The addition of eggs and cheese (or vegan alternatives) adds protein and calcium, making these breadsticks not only a tasty side or snack but also nutritionally beneficial. This recipe is ideal for those following a ketogenic or gluten-free diet, offering the comforting taste and texture of garlic bread without the carbs.

33. Marinated Artichoke Hearts

Prep time: 10 minutes (plus marinating time)

Serving size: 4 servings

Ingredients:

- 2 cups canned artichoke hearts, drained

- 1/4 cup olive oil

- 2 tablespoons lemon juice

- 2 cloves garlic, minced

- 1 teaspoon dried oregano

- 1/2 teaspoon red pepper flakes (adjust to taste)

- Salt and pepper to taste

- Fresh parsley, chopped, for garnish

Nutritional facts (per serving):

- Calories: 150 kcal

- Carbohydrates: 8g

- Fiber: 4g

- Protein: 2g

- Fat: 12g

Preparation directions:

1. In a bowl, whisk together the olive oil, lemon juice, minced garlic, dried oregano, red pepper flakes, salt, and pepper to create the marinade.
2. Add the drained artichoke hearts to the marinade, tossing gently to ensure they are well coated.
3. Cover and refrigerate for at least 2 hours, preferably overnight, allowing the flavors to meld.
4. Serve the marinated artichoke hearts garnished with fresh parsley. They can be enjoyed as a snack on their own or added to salads for extra flavor.

Health benefit:

Marinated Artichoke Hearts are a delicious and nutritious snack or side dish, offering several health benefits. Artichokes are a great source of fiber, which aids in digestion and helps to keep you feeling full longer. They also contain antioxidants like vitamin C and quercetin, which can protect the body from oxidative stress and support immune health. The olive oil in the marinade provides healthy fats that are beneficial for heart health. This dish is not only flavorful but also supports a balanced, healthy diet.

34. Roasted Brussels Sprouts with Pecans

Prep time: 10 minutes
Cook time: 20 minutes
Serving size: 4 servings

Ingredients:

- 1 pound Brussels sprouts, trimmed and halved

- 1/2 cup pecans, roughly chopped

- 2 tablespoons olive oil

- 1/2 teaspoon sea salt

- 1/4 teaspoon black pepper

- Balsamic glaze for drizzling (optional)

Nutritional facts (per serving):

- Calories: 180 kcal

- Carbohydrates: 10g

- Fiber: 4g

- Protein: 5g

- Fat: 14g

Preparation directions:

1. Preheat the oven to 400°F (200°C). Line a baking sheet with parchment paper.
2. In a large bowl, toss the Brussels sprouts and pecans with olive oil, salt, and pepper until well coated.
3. Spread the Brussels sprouts and pecans in a single layer on the prepared baking sheet.
4. Roast in the preheated oven for 20 minutes, or until the Brussels sprouts are tender and caramelized, stirring halfway through.
5. Drizzle with balsamic glaze before serving, if desired.

Health benefit:

Roasted Brussels Sprouts with Pecans is a hearty and healthful side dish packed with nutrients. Brussels sprouts are high in vitamins K and C, which support bone health and immune function, and contain compounds that may have antioxidant properties. Pecans add a crunchy texture and are a good source of healthy fats, magnesium, and fiber, contributing to heart health and digestion. This dish combines the nutritional benefits of both ingredients, making it a flavorful addition to any meal that supports overall health.

35. Eggplant Dip (Baba Ganoush)

Prep time: 15 minutes

Cook time: 45 minutes

Serving size: 4 servings

Ingredients:

- 2 medium eggplants

- 3 tablespoons tahini

- 2 cloves garlic, minced

- 2 tablespoons lemon juice

- 1 tablespoon olive oil

- 1/2 teaspoon ground cumin

- Salt to taste

- Fresh parsley, chopped, for garnish

- Paprika, for sprinkling

Nutritional facts (per serving):

- Calories: 140 kcal

- Carbohydrates: 13g

- Fiber: 6g

- Protein: 4g

- Fat: 9g

Preparation directions:

1. Preheat the oven to 400°F (200°C). Prick the eggplants with a fork and place them on a baking sheet.
2. Roast the eggplants in the oven for about 45 minutes, or until the skin is charred and the inside is tender.
3. Remove from the oven and let cool. Peel the skin off the eggplants and place the flesh in a colander to drain excess liquid.
4. In a food processor, combine the eggplant flesh, tahini, garlic, lemon juice, olive oil, cumin, and salt. Process until smooth.
5. Transfer the baba ganoush to a serving dish. Garnish with chopped parsley and a sprinkle of paprika.
6. Serve with low-carb vegetables or keto-friendly crackers for dipping.

Health benefit:

Eggplant Dip, or Baba Ganoush, is a flavorful and nutritious choice for a snack or side dish. Eggplant is low in calories but rich in fiber, vitamins, and minerals, including vitamin C, potassium, and manganese, which support heart health and blood pressure regulation. Tahini adds a creamy texture and is a good source of healthy fats, calcium, and antioxidants. This dip is not only delicious but also provides a variety of health benefits, making it a great addition to a low-carb, vegetarian diet.

36. Vegan Cheese (Nut-Based)

Prep time: 15 minutes (plus soaking time for nuts)
Serving size: 8 servings

Ingredients:

- 1 cup raw cashews, soaked for 4 hours or overnight, then drained

- 1/4 cup nutritional yeast

- 1 clove garlic

- 2 tablespoons lemon juice

- 1/2 teaspoon salt

- 1/4 teaspoon turmeric (for color)

- 1/2 cup water (or as needed for blending)

Nutritional facts (per serving):

- Calories: 130 kcal

- Carbohydrates: 8g

- Fiber: 1g

- Protein: 5g

- Fat: 10g

Preparation directions:

1. Place the soaked and drained cashews in a high-speed blender or food processor.
2. Add the nutritional yeast, garlic, lemon juice, salt, turmeric, and half of the water to start.
3. Blend on high until smooth and creamy, adding more water as needed to reach your desired consistency.
4. Taste and adjust seasoning as needed, adding more salt or lemon juice if desired.
5. Transfer the vegan cheese to a container and refrigerate until firm, about 2 hours, or serve immediately as a creamy spread.

Health benefit:

Vegan Cheese made from cashews is a nutritious and flavorful alternative to dairy cheese, suitable for a low-carb vegetarian diet. Cashews are a good source of healthy fats, magnesium, and zinc, which support brain health, immune function, and skin health. Nutritional yeast adds a cheesy flavor and is rich in B vitamins, including vitamin B12, essential for energy metabolism and nervous system health. This nut-based cheese is not only delicious but also offers a variety of health benefits, making it a versatile addition to snacks and meals.

37. Spicy Pumpkin Seeds

Prep time: 5 minutes

Cook time: 20 minutes

Serving size: 4 servings

Ingredients:

- 1 cup raw pumpkin seeds

- 1 tablespoon olive oil

- 1/2 teaspoon smoked paprika

- 1/4 teaspoon cayenne pepper (adjust to taste)

- Salt to taste

Nutritional facts (per serving):

- Calories: 180 kcal

- Carbohydrates: 3g

- Fiber: 1g

- Protein: 9g

- Fat: 16g

Preparation directions:

1. Preheat the oven to 350°F (175°C). Line a baking sheet with parchment paper.

2. In a bowl, toss the pumpkin seeds with olive oil, smoked paprika, cayenne pepper, and salt until well coated.

3. Spread the seasoned pumpkin seeds in a single layer on the prepared baking sheet.

4. Roast in the preheated oven for about 20 minutes, stirring occasionally, until the seeds are golden and crispy.

5. Let cool before serving. These can be enjoyed as a snack on their own or sprinkled over salads for added crunch and flavor.

Health benefit:

Spicy Pumpkin Seeds are a nutritious and savory snack that offers multiple health benefits. Pumpkin seeds are a great source of magnesium, zinc, and healthy fats, which contribute to heart health, immune function, and mood regulation. The spices not only add flavor but also contain antioxidants and anti-inflammatory properties. This snack is rich in protein and fiber, helping to promote satiety and support digestive health. Enjoying spicy pumpkin seeds is a delicious way to incorporate more nutrients into your diet while satisfying your craving for something savory.

38. Zucchini Chips

Prep time: 10 minutes

Cook time: 2 hours

Serving size: 4 servings

Ingredients:

- 2 large zucchinis, thinly sliced

- 1 tablespoon olive oil

- Salt to taste

- Optional seasonings: garlic powder, smoked paprika, or nutritional yeast

Nutritional facts (per serving):

- Calories: 60 kcal

- Carbohydrates: 4g

- Fiber: 1g

- Protein: 2g

- Fat: 4g

Preparation directions:

1. Preheat the oven to 225°F (105°C). Line several baking sheets with parchment paper.

2. In a bowl, toss the thinly sliced zucchini with olive oil and salt, ensuring each slice is lightly coated. Add any additional seasonings as desired.

3. Arrange the zucchini slices in a single layer on the prepared baking sheets, ensuring they do not overlap.

4. Bake in the preheated oven for 1.5 to 2 hours, flipping the slices halfway through, until they are crispy and lightly golden.

5. Let the chips cool on the baking sheets to crisp up further before serving.

Health benefit:

Zucchini Chips are a healthy, low-carb snack that offers a good source of vitamins A and C, potassium, and antioxidants. Zucchini is low in calories and high in water content, making these chips a hydrating and nutritious alternative to traditional fried snacks. The olive oil provides healthy monounsaturated fats, which are beneficial for heart health. These chips are a tasty way to increase vegetable intake, offering a crispy texture and flavor that can be customized with various seasonings.

39. Olive and Tomato Tapenade

Prep time: 10 minutes

Serving size: 4 servings

Ingredients:

- 1 cup pitted Kalamata olives

- 1/2 cup sun-dried tomatoes, drained if oil-packed

- 2 tablespoons capers, rinsed

- 2 cloves garlic

- 2 tablespoons olive oil

- 1 tablespoon lemon juice

- Fresh basil leaves, for garnish

Nutritional facts (per serving):

- Calories: 140 kcal

- Carbohydrates: 8g

- Fiber: 2g

- Protein: 1g

- Fat: 12g

Preparation directions:

1. In a food processor, combine the Kalamata olives, sun-dried tomatoes, capers, and garlic. Pulse until coarsely chopped.

2. With the processor running, slowly add the olive oil and lemon juice, processing until the mixture reaches your desired consistency.

3. Transfer the tapenade to a serving bowl and garnish with fresh basil leaves.

4. Serve with low-carb crackers or vegetable sticks for dipping.

Health benefit:

Olive and Tomato Tapenade is a flavorful and nutrient-dense snack or appetizer. Olives are rich in heart-healthy monounsaturated fats and antioxidants, which can help reduce inflammation and lower the risk of chronic diseases. Sun-dried tomatoes provide vitamins C and K, iron, and lycopene, an antioxidant with potential health benefits. This tapenade is a delicious way to enjoy a variety of nutrients while adding bold flavors to your meals and snacks.

40. Creamy Cucumber Salad with Dill

Prep time: 10 minutes

Serving size: 4 servings

Ingredients:

- 2 large cucumbers, thinly sliced

- 1/2 cup Greek yogurt (use dairy-free yogurt for vegan option)

- 2 tablespoons fresh dill, chopped

- 1 tablespoon lemon juice

- 1 clove garlic, minced

- Salt and pepper to taste

Nutritional facts (per serving):

- Calories: 50 kcal

- Carbohydrates: 6g

- Fiber: 1g

- Protein: 3g

- Fat: 2g

Preparation directions:

1. In a large bowl, combine the thinly sliced cucumbers, Greek yogurt, chopped dill, lemon juice, and minced garlic. Stir gently to combine.
2. Season with salt and pepper to taste.
3. Chill in the refrigerator for at least 30 minutes before serving to allow the flavors to meld.
4. Serve the creamy cucumber salad as a refreshing side dish, perfect for pairing with any meal.

Health benefit:

Creamy Cucumber Salad with Dill is a light and hydrating side dish, ideal for a low-carb diet. Cucumbers are rich in water content and provide a modest amount of vitamins K and C, which support hydration, skin health, and immune function. Greek yogurt adds a creamy texture and is a good source of protein and probiotics, promoting digestive health and muscle maintenance. Dill contributes to the dish's flavor and offers additional vitamins and minerals. This salad is a delightful and nutritious choice for adding freshness and hydration to your meals.

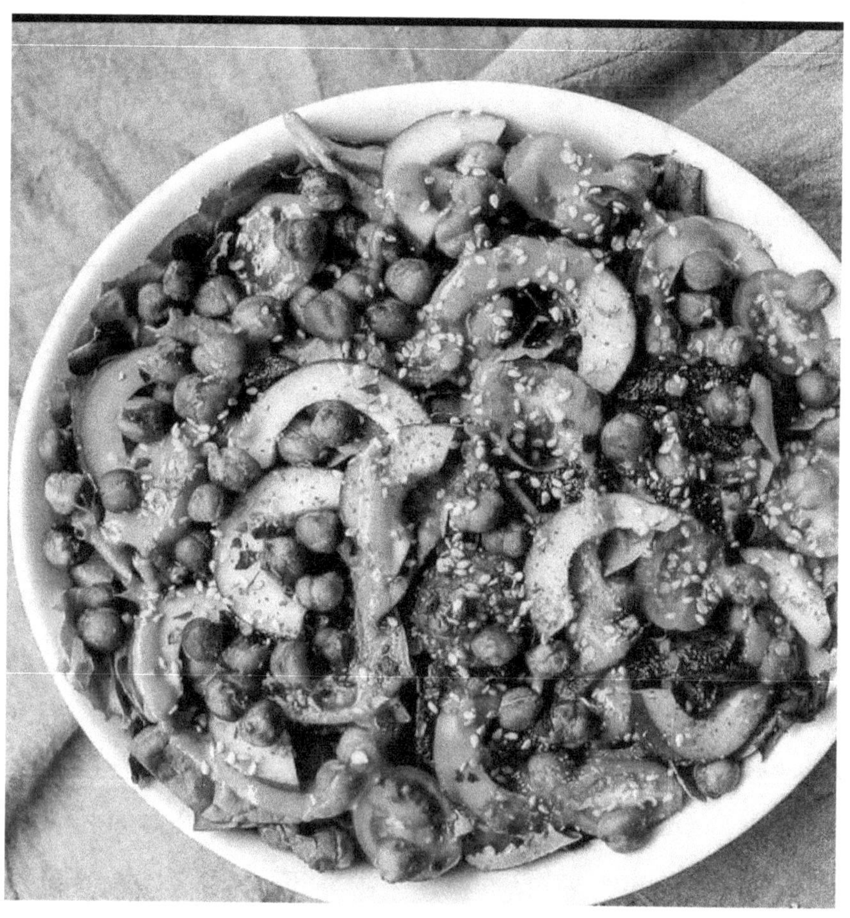

41. Blackberry and Mint Infused Water

Prep time: 5 minutes

Cook time: 0 minutes (Infuse for at least 2 hours)

Serving size: 4 servings

Ingredients:

- 4 cups water

- 1 cup fresh blackberries

- 1/4 cup fresh mint leaves

- Ice cubes, for serving

Nutritional facts (per serving):

- Calories: 10 kcal

- Carbohydrates: 2g

- Fiber: 1g

- Protein: 0g

- Fat: 0g

Preparation directions:

1. In a large pitcher, combine the water, fresh blackberries, and mint leaves.

2. Use a spoon to gently muddle the blackberries and mint leaves to release their flavors.

3. Refrigerate the pitcher for at least 2 hours, allowing the water to become infused with the flavors of the blackberries and mint.

4. Serve the infused water over ice cubes, garnishing with additional blackberries and mint leaves if desired.

Health benefit:

Blackberry and Mint Infused Water is a refreshing and hydrating drink that offers several health benefits. Blackberries are rich in antioxidants, vitamins C and K, and fiber, which can help support immune function, skin health, and digestion. Mint adds a refreshing flavor and has been linked to improved digestion and relief from nausea. This infused water is a delightful way to increase your daily water intake, promoting overall hydration and well-being without added sugars.

42. Coconut and Raspberry Keto Fat

Prep time: 10 minutes

Cook time: 0 minutes (Freeze for at least 1 hour)

Serving size: 12 fat bombs

Ingredients:

- 1 cup coconut oil, melted

- 1/2 cup unsweetened shredded coconut

- 1/2 cup fresh raspberries

- 1/4 cup almond flour

- 2 tablespoons erythritol (or other sugar-free sweetener)

- 1 teaspoon vanilla extract

Nutritional facts (per fat bomb):

- Calories: 150 kcal

- Carbohydrates: 2g

- Fiber: 1g

- Protein: 1g

- Fat: 16g

Preparation directions:

1. In a mixing bowl, combine the melted coconut oil, shredded coconut, almond flour, erythritol, and vanilla extract. Mix well until fully combined.
2. Gently fold in the fresh raspberries, being careful not to crush them.
3. Spoon the mixture into silicone molds or mini muffin cups.
4. Freeze for at least 1 hour, or until the fat bombs are solid.
5. Once solid, remove the fat bombs from the molds and store them in an airtight container in the freezer.

Health benefit:

Coconut and Raspberry Keto Fat Bombs are a delicious, energy-dense snack that supports a low-carb, high-fat diet. Coconut oil is rich in medium-chain triglycerides (MCTs), which can help increase energy expenditure and promote satiety. Raspberries add natural sweetness, antioxidants, and fiber with minimal carbs. Almond flour provides additional healthy fats and vitamin E, an antioxidant important for skin health. These fat bombs are perfect for satisfying sweet cravings while adhering to ketogenic dietary guidelines, offering a nutritious snack or dessert option.

43. Almond Butter and Chocolate Fudge

Prep time: 10 minutes
Cook time: 0 minutes (Chill for at least 2 hours)
Serving size: 16 pieces

Ingredients:

- 1 cup almond butter

- 1/2 cup coconut oil

- 1/4 cup unsweetened cocoa powder

- 1/4 cup sugar-free sweetener (e.g., erythritol or monk fruit sweetener)

- 1 teaspoon vanilla extract

- A pinch of salt

Nutritional facts (per piece):

- Calories: 150 kcal

- Carbohydrates: 4g

- Fiber: 2g

- Protein: 4g

- Fat: 14g

Preparation directions:

1. In a medium saucepan over low heat, melt the coconut oil and almond butter together, stirring until smooth.

2. Remove from heat and whisk in the cocoa powder, sweetener, vanilla extract, and a pinch of salt until well combined and smooth.

3. Pour the mixture into a lined 8x8 inch baking dish or silicone mold.

4. Refrigerate for at least 2 hours, or until the fudge is firm.

5. Cut into 16 pieces and serve. Store any leftovers in the refrigerator.

Health benefit:

Almond Butter and Chocolate Fudge is a rich and satisfying dessert that fits well within a low-carb or ketogenic diet. Almond butter provides a good source of protein, healthy fats, and fiber, contributing to satiety and supporting heart health. Coconut oil contains MCTs, which may support weight management and metabolic health. Unsweetened cocoa powder adds antioxidants without extra sugar, offering mood-boosting benefits. This dessert is a guilt-free way to enjoy the decadence of fudge while maintaining nutritional goals.

44. Lemon Cheesecake Mousse (Sugar-Free)

Prep time: 15 minutes
Cook time: 0 minutes (Chill for at least 1 hour)
Serving size: 4 servings

Ingredients:

- 8 oz cream cheese, softened (use dairy-free cream cheese for vegan option)
- 1/2 cup heavy cream (use coconut cream for vegan option)
- 1/4 cup sugar-free sweetener (e.g., erythritol or monk fruit sweetener)

- 2 tablespoons lemon juice
- 1 teaspoon lemon zest
- 1 teaspoon vanilla extract

Nutritional facts (per serving):

- Calories: 250 kcal

- Carbohydrates: 3g

- Fiber: 0g

- Protein: 4g

- Fat: 25g

Preparation directions:

1. In a large mixing bowl, beat the cream cheese until smooth.

2. Add the heavy cream (or coconut cream) and beat until the mixture starts to thicken.

3. Gradually beat in the sweetener, lemon juice, lemon zest, and vanilla extract until well combined and the mixture is light and fluffy.

4. Divide the mousse into serving dishes and refrigerate for at least 1 hour to set.

5. Garnish with additional lemon zest before serving, if desired.

Health benefit:

Lemon Cheesecake Mousse provides a light and refreshing dessert option that is low in carbohydrates and sugar-free, making it suitable for those following a ketogenic or low-carb diet. Cream cheese and heavy cream (or their vegan alternatives) offer a rich source of healthy fats, contributing to a creamy texture and a sense of satiety. Lemon juice and zest add a burst of flavor as well as vitamin C, an antioxidant that supports immune health. This dessert is a delightful way to end a meal or enjoy a treat without impacting blood sugar levels.

45. Strawberries Dipped in Vegan Dark Chocolate

Prep time: 15 minutes
Cook time: 5 minutes (Plus chilling time)
Serving size: 4 servings

Ingredients:

- 1 cup vegan dark chocolate chips

- 1 tablespoon coconut oil

- 16 fresh strawberries, washed and dried

- Optional toppings: chopped nuts, shredded coconut, or sea salt

Nutritional facts (per serving):

- Calories: 220 kcal

- Carbohydrates: 25g

- Fiber: 3g

- Protein: 2g

- Fat: 14g

Preparation directions:

1. In a microwave-safe bowl, combine the vegan dark chocolate chips and coconut oil. Microwave in 30-second intervals, stirring between each, until the chocolate is fully melted and smooth.

2. Holding the strawberries by the stem, dip each one into the melted chocolate, letting the excess drip off.

3. Place the dipped strawberries on a parchment-lined tray. Sprinkle with optional toppings if desired.

4. Chill the strawberries in the refrigerator until the chocolate sets, about 30 minutes.

5. Serve the chocolate-dipped strawberries as a decadent yet healthy dessert or snack.

Health benefit:

Strawberries Dipped in Vegan Dark Chocolate is a simple and elegant dessert that combines the health benefits of dark chocolate with the nutritional goodness of strawberries. Dark chocolate is rich in antioxidants, such as flavonoids, which may improve heart health and reduce inflammation. Strawberries are a great source of vitamin C, manganese, and fiber, supporting immune function and digestive health. This dessert offers a delightful way to enjoy the benefits of fruit and dark chocolate in a form that's both indulgent and health-conscious.

46. Matcha Chia Seed Pudding

Prep time: 10 minutes

Cook time: 0 minutes (Refrigerate for at least 4 hours or overnight)

Serving size: 4 servings

Ingredients:

- 1/4 cup chia seeds

- 1 cup unsweetened almond milk

- 1 cup coconut milk

- 2 tablespoons sugar-free sweetener (e.g., erythritol or monk fruit sweetener)

- 1 teaspoon matcha green tea powder

- 1/2 teaspoon vanilla extract

Nutritional facts (per serving):

- Calories: 180 kcal

- Carbohydrates: 8g

- Fiber: 6g

- Protein: 4g

- Fat: 14g

Preparation directions:

1. In a bowl, whisk together the almond milk, coconut milk, sweetener, matcha powder, and vanilla extract until well combined and the matcha is fully dissolved.

2. Stir in the chia seeds until evenly distributed.

3. Divide the mixture among serving glasses or bowls. Cover and refrigerate for at least 4 hours, or overnight, until the pudding has thickened and the chia seeds have absorbed the liquid.

4. Before serving, give the pudding a stir and adjust the sweetness if necessary. Garnish with a sprinkle of matcha powder or fresh fruit, if desired.

Health benefit:

Matcha Chia Seed Pudding is a nutritious and energizing dessert or snack option. Chia seeds are a great source of omega-3 fatty acids, fiber, and protein, supporting heart health, digestion, and satiety.

Matcha green tea powder provides a unique blend of antioxidants, particularly EGCG (epigallocatechin gallate), which has been linked to numerous health benefits, including improved metabolism and a reduced risk of heart disease. This pudding combines the healthful properties of chia seeds and matcha, making it a perfect choice for a health-conscious treat that also provides a gentle caffeine boost.

47. Pumpkin Pie Smoothie (Dairy-Free)

Prep time: 5 minutes
Serving size: 2 servings

Ingredients:
- 1 cup pumpkin puree (not pumpkin pie filling)
- 1 1/2 cups almond milk (or any dairy-free milk)
- 1/2 banana, frozen
- 2 tablespoons sugar-free sweetener (e.g., erythritol or monk fruit sweetener)
- 1 teaspoon pumpkin pie spice
- 1/2 teaspoon vanilla extract
- Ice cubes, as needed

Nutritional facts (per serving):

- Calories: 100 kcal

- Carbohydrates: 18g

- Fiber: 5g

- Protein: 2g

- Fat: 2g

Preparation directions:

1. In a blender, combine the pumpkin puree, almond milk, frozen banana, sweetener, pumpkin pie spice, vanilla extract, and ice cubes.
2. Blend on high until smooth and creamy, adjusting the amount of ice to achieve your desired consistency.
3. Taste and adjust the sweetness or spices if necessary.
4. Pour the smoothie into glasses and serve immediately, garnished with a sprinkle of pumpkin pie spice or cinnamon, if desired.

Health benefit:

Pumpkin Pie Smoothie offers a dairy-free, low-carb treat that captures the essence of fall flavors while providing nutritional benefits. Pumpkin puree is high in vitamins A and C, potassium, and fiber, supporting immune health, vision, and digestion. The addition of banana provides natural sweetness and additional fiber, while almond milk offers a light, dairy-free base rich in vitamin E. This smoothie is a delightful way to enjoy the taste of pumpkin pie in a healthier, drinkable form.

48. Keto Avocado Popsicles

Prep time: 10 minutes
Cook time: 0 minutes (Freeze for at least 4 hours)
Serving size: 6 popsicles

Ingredients:

- 2 ripe avocados

- 1 cup coconut milk

- 1/4 cup lime juice

- 1/4 cup sugar-free sweetener (e.g., erythritol or monk fruit sweetener)

- 1/2 teaspoon vanilla extract

- Pinch of salt

Nutritional facts (per popsicle):

- Calories: 150 kcal

- Carbohydrates: 8g

- Fiber: 4g

- Protein: 2g

- Fat: 13g

Preparation directions:

1. Scoop the avocado flesh into a blender. Add the coconut milk, lime juice, sweetener, vanilla extract, and a pinch of salt.
2. Blend until smooth and creamy, with no lumps remaining.
3. Pour the mixture into popsicle molds, inserting sticks according to the mold's instructions.
4. Freeze for at least 4 hours, or until fully set.
5. To release the popsicles, run warm water over the outside of the molds for a few seconds.
6. Serve the avocado popsicles as a refreshing and keto-friendly dessert.

Health benefit:

Keto Avocado Popsicles are a creamy and satisfying treat perfect for a low-carb diet. Avocados provide healthy fats, fiber, and essential nutrients like potassium and vitamin E, supporting heart health and skin integrity. Coconut milk adds richness and a source of medium-chain triglycerides (MCTs), which may aid in weight management and energy levels. Lime juice offers a burst of vitamin C and antioxidants. These popsicles are a fantastic way to indulge in a sweet, frozen treat without straying from ketogenic nutritional goals.

49. Cinnamon and Pecan Porridge (Flaxseed Meal)

Prep time: 5 minutes

Cook time: 5 minutes

Serving size: 2 servings

Ingredients:

- 1/2 cup flaxseed meal

- 1 cup almond milk (or any dairy-free milk)

- 2 tablespoons chopped pecans

- 1 tablespoon sugar-free sweetener (e.g., erythritol or monk fruit sweetener)

- 1/2 teaspoon cinnamon

- Pinch of salt

Nutritional facts (per serving):

- Calories: 220 kcal

- Carbohydrates: 8g

- Fiber: 7g

- Protein: 6g

- Fat: 18g

Preparation directions:

1. In a small saucepan, combine the flaxseed meal, almond milk, sweetener, cinnamon, and a pinch of salt. Stir well to mix.
2. Cook over medium heat, stirring frequently, until the mixture thickens to a porridge-like consistency, about 3-5 minutes.
3. Remove from heat and divide the porridge between two bowls.
4. Top with chopped pecans and an additional sprinkle of cinnamon before serving.

Health benefit:

Cinnamon and Pecan Porridge made with flaxseed meal is a nutritious, low-carb breakfast option that provides a wealth of health benefits. Flaxseed is rich in omega-3 fatty acids, lignans, and fiber, promoting heart health, hormonal balance, and digestive well-being. Cinnamon adds natural sweetness and has been linked to blood sugar regulation. Pecans contribute healthy fats, protein, and antioxidants. This warm and comforting porridge is an excellent way to start the day, offering sustained energy and essential nutrients.

50. Ginger and Lemon Hot Tea (Sweetened with Stevia)

Prep time: 5 minutes

Cook time: 10 minutes

Serving size: 2 servings

Ingredients:

- 4 cups water

- 2 inches fresh ginger, peeled and thinly sliced

- 1/2 lemon, juiced

- Stevia to taste

- Lemon slices and fresh ginger slices, for garnish

Nutritional facts (per serving):

- Calories: 10 kcal

- Carbohydrates: 3g

- Fiber: 0g

- Protein: 0g

- Fat: 0g

Preparation directions:

1. In a medium saucepan, bring the water to a boil. Add the sliced ginger to the boiling water.

2. Reduce the heat and simmer for 10 minutes to allow the ginger to infuse.

3. Remove from heat and stir in the lemon juice. Sweeten with stevia to taste.

4. Strain the tea into cups, discarding the ginger slices.

5. Garnish each cup with a slice of lemon and a slice of fresh ginger, if desired.

Health benefit:

Ginger and Lemon Hot Tea sweetened with stevia is a soothing and healthful drink that provides numerous benefits. Ginger is well-known for its anti-inflammatory properties and its ability to alleviate nausea and digestive issues. Lemon juice adds vitamin C and enhances the immune system, while stevia provides a natural, zero-calorie sweetness. This tea is an ideal choice for warming up on a cold day or for settling the stomach after a meal, offering a comforting, health-promoting beverage without added sugars.

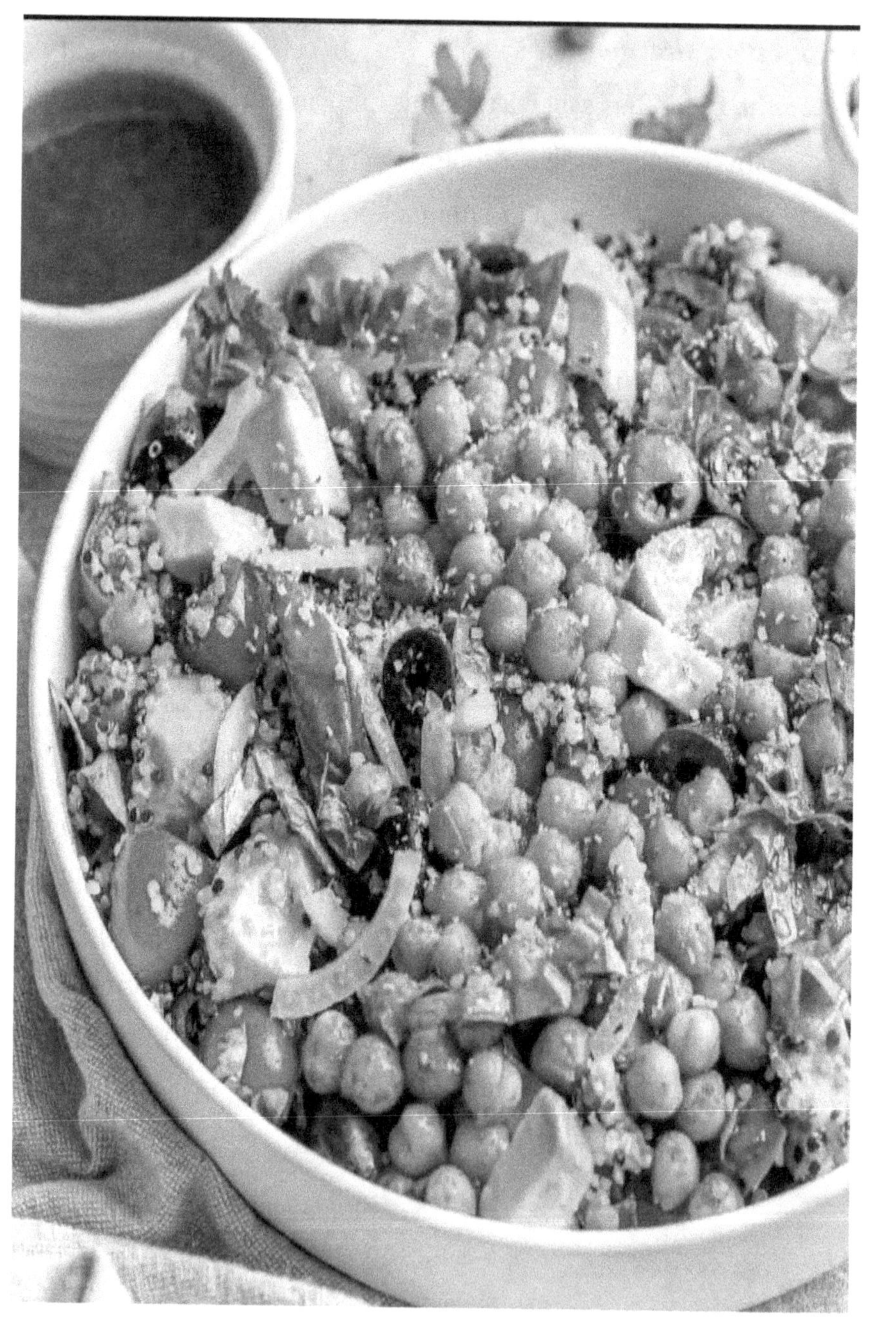

CHAPTER 6: 14-DAY LOW-CARB VEGETARIAN MEAL PLAN

Embarking on a low-carb vegetarian diet can be both exciting and daunting. To ease this transition and help you maintain this lifestyle, we've crafted a comprehensive 14-day meal plan. This plan integrates recipes from our cookbook, providing a balanced, nutritious, and varied diet that adheres to low-carb principles while satisfying your vegetarian preferences. Each day includes three meals—breakfast, lunch, and dinner—designed to fuel your body and delight your taste buds without the guesswork.

Day 1
- Breakfast: Chia and Almond Milk Porridge (#1)
- Lunch: Zucchini Noodles with Avocado Pesto (#11)
- Dinner: Mushroom Stroganoff (Zucchini Noodles) (#21)

Day 2
- Breakfast: Low-Carb Blueberry Muffins (Almond Flour) (#4)
- Lunch: Greek Salad with Tofu Feta (#14)
- Dinner: Cauliflower Steak with Chimichurri Sauce (#22)

Day 3

- Breakfast: Keto Avocado Smoothie with Coconut Milk (#3)

- Lunch: Creamy Spinach Soup (Dairy-Free) (#13)

- Dinner: Baked Tofu with Peanut Sauce and Stir-Fry Veggies (#24)

Day 4

- Breakfast: Spinach and Mushroom Omelet Cups (#2)

- Lunch: Caprese Stuffed Avocado (#15)

- Dinner: Spaghetti Squash with Creamy Mushroom Sauce (#23)

Day 5

- Breakfast: Shakshuka with Feta (No Bread) (#5)

- Lunch: Cauliflower Tabouleh (#12)

- Dinner: Grilled Halloumi with Mediterranean Vegetables (#25)

Day 6

- Breakfast: Pumpkin Spice Chia Pudding (#10)

- Lunch: Roasted Red Pepper and Goat Cheese Zucchini Rolls (#20)

- Dinner: Vegan Alfredo with Shirataki Noodles (#26)

Day 7

- Breakfast: Bell Pepper and Kale Frittata (#9)

- Lunch: Broccoli and Almond Salad (#16)

- Dinner: Paneer Tikka Skewers (#29)

Day 8

- Breakfast: Almond and Flaxseed Pancakes (#7)

- Lunch: Keto Eggplant Pizza Rounds (#17)

- Dinner: Stuffed Bell Peppers (Quinoa and Vegetables) (#28)

Day 9

- Breakfast: Coconut Yogurt with Nuts and Seeds (#8)

- Lunch: Cucumber Boat with Spicy Tofu Salad (#18)

- Dinner: Moroccan Tagine with Turnip and Zucchini (#30)

Day 10

- Breakfast: Almond Flour Pancakes (#1) - Use a different recipe
to avoid repetition, such as Coconut Chia Pudding (#4)

- Lunch: Asparagus and Artichoke Heart Salad (#19)

- Dinner: Vegetable Korma (Cauliflower Rice) (#27)

Day 11

- Breakfast: Low-Carb Berry Smoothie (#5)–Use a different recipe to avoid repetition, such as Flaxseed and Walnut Porridge (#6)
- Lunch: Greek Salad with Tofu Feta (#14)–Repeat for variety and simplicity.
- Dinner: Baked Ratatouille with Mozzarella (#29)–Use a different recipe to avoid repetition, such as Spaghetti Squash Alfredo with Spinach (#27)

Day 12

- Breakfast: Cauliflower and Cheese Breakfast Muffins (#6)–Use a different recipe for variety, such as Keto Avocado Smoothie with Coconut Milk (#3)
- Lunch: Egg Salad with Avocado (#14)–Modify to a different lunch recipe for variety, such as Stuffed Avocados with Cottage Cheese and Nuts (#13)
- Dinner: Vegan Shepherd's Pie with Cauliflower Mash (#30)–Adjust to another dinner recipe for diversity, like Eggplant Parmesan (Baked, No Breading) (#21)

Day 13

- Breakfast: Pumpkin Spice Chia Pudding (#10)–Repeat for ease and enjoyment.
- Lunch: Broccoli and Cheddar Soup (#19)–Change to a different recipe for variety, such as Creamy Spinach Soup (Dairy-Free) (#13)
- Dinner: Paneer Tikka Masala (#28)–Adjust to a different recipe for new flavors, such as Cauliflower Fried Rice (#18)

Day 14

- Breakfast: Shakshuka with Feta (No Bread) (#5)–Repeat for a satisfying end to the two-week plan.
- Lunch: Avocado and Kale Salad with Lemon-Tahini Dressing (#20)–Use a different recipe for a fresh lunch option, like Cauliflower Rice Salad with Lemon Dressing (#11)
- Dinner: Baked Zucchini Boats (#25)–Change to a different dinner option for the final night, such as Zucchini Lasagna (#23)

This meal plan is designed to introduce variety and ensure nutritional balance, offering a taste of the diverse flavors and ingredients that low-carb vegetarian cooking has to offer. Feel free to swap meals between days to suit your taste preferences and schedule, ensuring this diet remains enjoyable and sustainable.

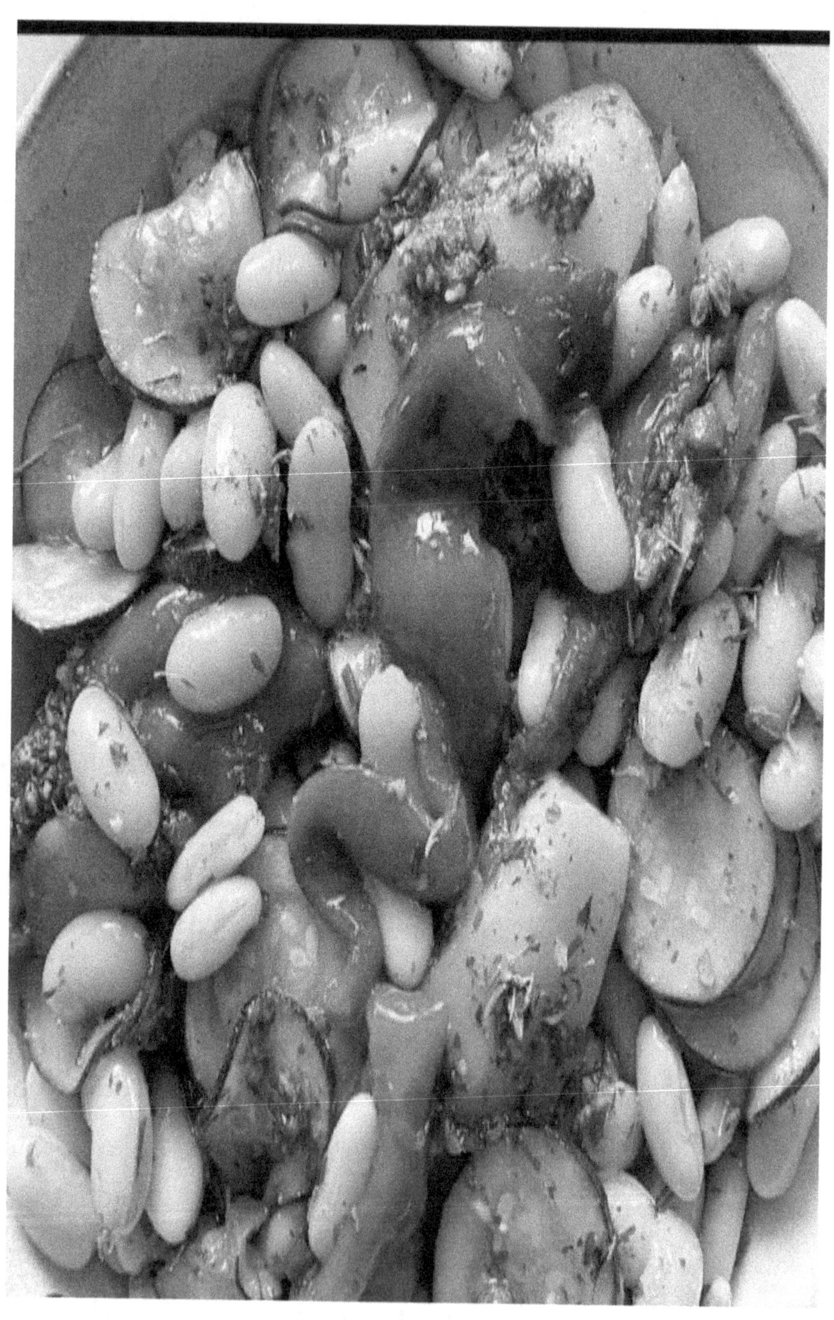

CONCLUSION

As you reach the end of this "Low-Carb Vegetarian Diet Cookbook for Beginners," it's important to recognize that adopting a new dietary lifestyle is not just about following recipes but also about making sustainable changes that fit your personal health goals and preferences. The journey you've embarked on is highly personal and adaptable, and the key to long-term success lies in finding the right balance that works for you. Here are some tips and strategies to ensure your continued success on a low-carb vegetarian diet and how you can adapt and personalize recipes to meet your needs.

Tips for Long-Term Success on a Low-Carb Vegetarian Diet

1. Listen to Your Body: Pay attention to how different foods make you feel. Some people thrive on a higher intake of fats, while others may need more protein. Adjust your diet accordingly.

2. Keep Experimenting: The variety of low-carb vegetarian foods is vast. Don't be afraid to try new ingredients and cooking methods. This will keep your meals interesting and prevent dietary boredom.

3. Plan Your Meals: Planning ahead can help you avoid the temptation of off-plan eating. Use the 14-day meal plan as a template and continue to build your own meal plans as you become more comfortable with your dietary choices.

4. Stay Informed: Nutritional science evolves constantly. Stay informed about the latest research on low-carb vegetarian eating and adjust your diet to incorporate new findings and recommendations.

5. Seek Support: Whether it's joining online communities, finding a diet buddy, or consulting with a nutritionist, having support can make a significant difference in maintaining your dietary lifestyle.

How to Adapt and Personalize Recipes for Your Needs

1. Modifying Ingredients: If you have allergies, intolerances, or simply don't like certain ingredients, don't hesitate to substitute them. For example, if a recipe calls for nuts and you're allergic, try using seeds as an alternative.

2. Adjusting Macronutrients: Depending on your individual goals (e.g., weight loss, maintenance, muscle gain), you may need to adjust the macronutrient ratios of recipes. This could mean adding more protein sources like tofu or seitan to a dish or incorporating healthy fats through avocados or olive oil.

3. Experimenting with Flavors: Don't be afraid to change up the spices and herbs to suit your taste preferences. This can transform a dish without significantly impacting its nutritional profile.

4. Portion Control: Adjusting portion sizes can help you manage your caloric intake more effectively, depending on your specific goals. Use measuring tools and scales as needed to ensure accuracy.

5. Incorporating Local and Seasonal Produce: Take advantage of local and seasonal fruits and vegetables. Not only can this approach be more sustainable, but it can also introduce you to new flavors and nutrients.

Remember, the goal of "Low-Carb Vegetarian Diet Cookbook for Beginners" is to provide you with a foundation for healthy eating. As you grow more confident in your cooking and dietary choices, feel empowered to make the adjustments that best suit your lifestyle and preferences. Here's to a journey of health, discovery, and enjoyment on your low-carb vegetarian path.

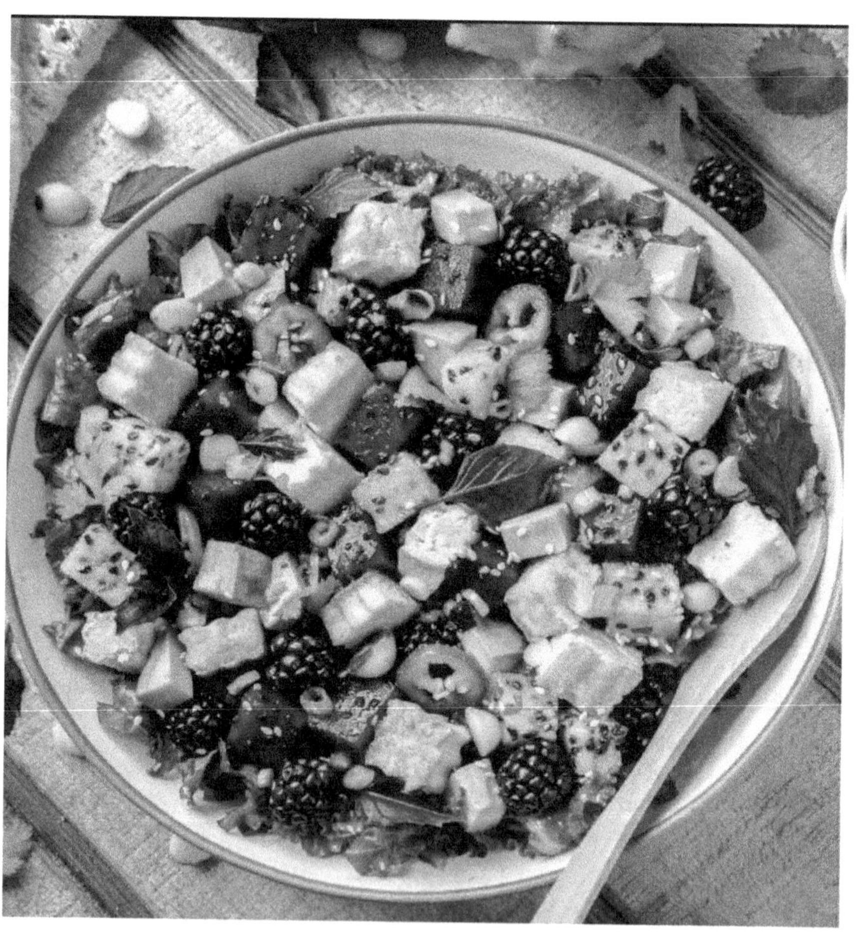